Strength
Training
on the
Ball

Also by Colleen Craig

Pilates on the Ball: The World's Most Popular Workout Using the Exercise Ball

Pilates on the Ball: A Comprehensive Book and DVD Workout

Abs on the Ball: A Pilates Approach to Building Superb Abdominals

Strength Training
on the
Ball

A Pilates Approach to Optimal
Strength and Balance

Colleen Craig

Healing Arts Press
Rochester, Vermont

Healing Arts Press
One Park Street
Rochester, Vermont 05767
www.InnerTraditions.com

Healing Arts Press is a division of Inner Traditions International

Note to the reader: This book is intended as an informational guide. The remedies, approaches, and techniques described herein are meant to supplement, and not to be a substitute for, professional medical care or treatment. They should not be used to treat a serious ailment without prior consultation with a qualified health care professional.

Library of Congress Cataloging-in-Publication Data
Craig, Colleen.
    Strength training on the ball : a pilates approach to optimal strength and balance / Colleen Craig.
        p. cm.
    ISBN 978-1-59477-011-1
    1. Pilates method. 2. Swiss exercise balls. I. Title.
    RA781.4.C73 2005
    613.7'1'0284—dc22

                                                                                            2005001934

Printed and bound in the United States

10 9 8 7 6 5 4 3

Photographs by David Scollard and Robert Barnett
Illustrations by Laraine Arsenault

Text design by Cindy Sutherland
Text layout by Virginia Scott Bowman
This book was typeset in Goudy with Avant Garde as the display typeface.

Contents

Introduction

Function Versus Strength

*If I were a Bengal tiger I
would hope my prey was big
on bulk and small on function.*
—Paul Chek, founder,
Corrective Holistic
Exercise Kinesiology

Liuda's Story

I set out for the outskirts of Moscow at midday. The subway was a standing-room-only crush. Elbows were loose; I felt one in my back. At one stop three market women squeezed in front of me and rolled their waist-high sack of potatoes over my toes.

I could not read the Russian signs so I began to count the stops on my fingers. My friend Liuda, short for Liudmila, lived in one of the sprawling, box-like Khrushchev-era apartment complexes in outer Moscow and I wondered what I would find when I arrived there. Liuda, sixty, had not left her flat once in five months. On a frigid December day the previous year, she fell on the ice and fractured her right hip.

I recalled the last time I saw her a couple of years back. After nearly three hours at her table, I was escorted back to the metro by Liuda, a recently retired yet youthful, indefatigable hostess. Now it was my turn to give back. A hip break at her age was dire. Statistics show that hip fractures in her age group and older can lead to loss of independence, a move to nursing homes, or even early deaths. Usually with hip fractures—especially femoral neck fractures such as Liuda had—surgery occurs in the first twenty-four to forty-eight hours after the injury and the goal of postoperative care is to get the patient up and moving as quickly as possible. This is not what had happened. Because her unlucky fall occurred so close to Russian New Year's Eve celebrations and drunk fêtes, she had to wait an unimaginable twenty days before an operation, her right leg kept immobile in a cast. After the operation—in which Liuda

1

had a pin inserted with a clang she could hear but not feel—she eventually returned to her apartment and had been homebound and chair bound since then. The only news I had from her was one long-distance call. Doctors "told her nothing," she said, and numerous friends who had never had hip operations "offered much advice." A friend, who had read somewhere that no movement could lead to blood clots and other complications, had given her a few exercises to do sitting on her bed. Since I was coming to Moscow for a holiday, Liuda asked me to look at the exercises she was now doing and add to these.

"Has the bone healed?" I had asked her the night before on the phone. Jet-lagged, disoriented by a sun that took forever to set and a phone that would click dead for no reason, I adjusted my ear to her accent. "Yes," she announced. "What is the word?—*consolidation*—is successful." This is what the young X-ray technician, who she paid in U.S. dollars to bring his machine to her place, had told her.

I got out at Liuda's subway stop and made my way past a gauntlet of hawkers and street vendors to the long path that weaved through an overgrown field to her apartment building. The path was scarred by deep potholes and guarded by an assortment of muddy stray dogs that would have given Red Riding Hood's wolf a fright. The stairs up to Liuda's flat were uneven, some of the tiles broken. I could see why she had not ventured out, but how had she coped with confining herself for five months to three small rooms? In addition, her doctor had instructed her by phone not to put any weight on her leg until he was able to examine her.

Over tea Liuda explained how she had devised a way to maneuver from one end of her apartment to the other. I didn't quite get it. She put her glass of tea down and demonstrated. I watched her hoist a wooden chair into the air and move it across her body to the other side. Then, using upper-body strength, she scooted herself across one chair seat to the other. It took her time, but she was able to get from her daybed in the front room down the hall to the bathroom and kitchen and back again.

The doctor soon arrived. He studied the X-ray and repeated in Russian what the technician had said the week before: "Everything is in order." He was a no-nonsense, Soviet-style man in his late fifties, but I got a small smile out of him as I flopped down on the mat I'd brought along and presented him with a series of exercises to determine what I should and should not do with Liuda. We agreed on a course of action and the doctor was on his way. A few minutes later so was I, after planning to meet Liuda in two days to begin the exercises.

That night I managed to find an old English dictionary in the Moscow apartment where I was staying. I had just begun writing on strength training using the ball and the Pilates Method, but Liuda's predicament brought my thoughts on this subject to a standstill. The dictionary defined *strength* as the capacity for exertion and the power to resist force. The image of a bodybuilder using raw effort and bulk to press a heavy weight into the air comes to mind. But what does this sort of muscular power have to do with other components of fitness: suppleness, speed, balance, aerobic health, and most important of all—function?

That evening I sat at the kitchen table and, using stick figures, drew out each of Liuda's exercises on yellow post-it notes. How many sessions per week and how many exercises per session were just two of the questions I asked myself. Like the guidebooks that I studied in the day to aid me in getting around Moscow, by night I studied the textbook photocopies on hip fractures that I had brought with me to help Liuda. Keeping the doctors dos and don'ts in mind, I moved the yellow post-its around on the table to decide what order would be easiest and most effective for Liuda—a generally healthy, pain free, nonexerciser—to follow.

As the Moscow twilight lingered past ten o'clock, the challenge ahead of me loomed large. Dictionary definitions of the words *function*, *strength*, and *endurance* lay scribbled on post-its beside the tic-tac-toe arrangement of the exercises. Luckily, the dictionary had also provided me with synonyms for *strength*: "solidity," "toughness," and "moral force." The reminder that strength equals moral fiber was encouraging. I knew Liuda possessed the resourcefulness and resolve typical of Russian women who have witnessed much change and adversity. In addition, even though she had never lifted a barbell in her life, she possessed some degree of muscular endurance from a life void of kitchen and other household conveniences. If not, this sixty-year-old woman would never have been able to heave solid wooden chairs around in the first place. But without specialized exercises to recover strength to her hip joints, legs, and buttock muscles, the future looked very bleak. Without resistance training, how would Liuda recover the balance and mobility to navigate smoothly from one point to another, not only through her small apartment but in the larger world?

Recovering Function and Strength

After working with Liuda (to whom we will return in the final chapter) and keeping in mind the considerable feedback I had received from my first two books, I made the decision that *Strength Training on the Ball* must cover much more than just weight training and the ball. Equally important is flexibility, abdominal strength, low-back-pain prevention, how to recover strength after

muscles and aging

Even without suffering a major trauma to the body, we lose muscle and strength at an alarming rate as we age. Some studies say the process begins in our early twenties; other studies say by age forty we lose muscle each year. This process is particularly significant for women, who tend to have smaller bodies and smaller bones and are not as used as men are to exerting their bodies against resistance.

If you don't use a muscle it weakens rapidly, as the NASA scientists discovered when the first men they sent up into space returned with significant muscle and strength loss. Why? The astronauts didn't use their muscles to get around in their weightless environment.

an injury, and the all-important posture and balance training. Most vital was that this book would be for all ages and levels of fitness. I wanted to show a progression of strength exercises, from those that are used for rehabilitation and low-back pain to exercises designed for total body conditioning and training.

Strength training is one of the key reasons most people give for going to a gym: men traditionally head for the mirrored weight-training section, women to the body sculpting classes. In North America millions of dollars a week are spent on personal trainers, gym memberships, strength-building magazines, books, videos, DVDs, and various nutritional supplements claiming to facilitate the growth of muscles. Though the goals and ultimate results vary considerably between men and women and from person to person, people take up strength training to deliberately change their bodies. Whether from personal vanity, competitive edge, or recovering from a serious injury like Liuda's, they desire strength, vigor, and change.

But what is the safest, most efficient way to embark on a strength-training program? At what point do raw strength and bulky, rigid muscles get in the way of function? And how do you ensure that the muscles are properly trained for your competition, recreational activity, or recovery?

One of the most exciting aspects of *Strength Training on the Ball* is the use of balls to target deep as well as superficial muscles and add resistance and weight bearing to mat exercises.

Exercise balls and free weights are versatile tools for manipulating the angle of your effort and working through a full range of motion. Working on the ball forces you to maintain your balance and center of gravity over a mobile base of support and allows you to work the body as a unit. The labile quality of the ball creates an unparalleled opportunity for balance training, a focus lacking in many programs. Better balance could mean the split-second adjustment that helps to prevent a fall or enable an athlete or dancer to better execute a challenging maneuver. Ball training develops strength and balance simultaneously—a much more functional way to train whether you are an older adult, core-weakened sedentary or postnatal woman, postoperative patient, teen, child, or elite athlete. You do not need to purchase a lot of equipment to get started. All you need is an exercise ball, a couple of sets of light free weights (1, 2, 3, and 5 pounds), and an elastic resistance band used for exercise. Resistance bands are about 5 feet long and $5\frac{1}{2}$ inches wide and color coded to let you know their degree of resistance. Tips for selecting the correct ball are at the end of chapter 2.

Connecting the Dots: A Pilates Approach

Sometimes recovering or enhancing strength is like being confronted with a series of dots in a child's picture. How does one proceed? Should we add a higher resistance or a different arc of movement? Do we place ourselves on a seated bench press so we can push more pounds or do we move ourselves onto an unstable surface where we will only lift a fraction of the weight but also use key postural and other stabilizing muscles? Do we trace in the lines with precision or scribble them in place with speed? And when the dots are finally connected together with the appropriate repetitions, sets, loads, and rest intervals, how can we know if we have produced a clear and effective movement pattern or a faulty and unintelligible one?

Correctly connecting the dots *within* the exercises and *between* the exercises was more important to Joseph H. Pilates than the number of repetitions or amount of weight lifted. Traditional strength training uses heavy weights to overload muscles by working them to fatigue and causing them to rebuild. A Pilates approach would take a bodybuilder off a weight machine and seat him or her on a ball or in a unique relationship to gravity using much lighter weights. This combination would get all parts of the body working together, not just the large muscles of the arms and chest.

A Pilates approach works the body from the inside out—a fundamental difference between this and other approaches. The small muscles deep inside the body are designed to provide support for the spine and the outer layer of musculature for maintaining postural integrity. The stronger this deep inner layer, the more efficiently the outer muscles can work without risk to the body. This approach keeps the muscles in balance and trains them properly for the jobs they are meant to do—an approach beneficial for men, women, children, and older populations as well as competitive and recreational athletes. The result is a body that feels taller and more poised and accomplishes tasks with ease and power.

Not a Recipe Book

Strength Training on the Ball is not simply a recipe book of exercises. The stories at the beginning of each chapter are meant to guide and inspire teachers and students alike, and the text that follows will provide you with important information to understand how your body functions. Perhaps you are like many of us and need to make a radical change in your life to incorporate a fitness routine. The check-ins at the end of each chapter vary in topics from

physical versus mental strength

What is the link between physical strength, mental strength, and confidence? Jan Todd, one of the world's strongest women and a historian of women's strength training at the University of Texas in Austin, describes how physical fragility can lead to a lack of confidence in other parts of one's life. "I see friends in their forties pushing away from life, not trying things," said Todd, adding, "the physicality of my life taught me not to be afraid."

Jake Steinfeld of the famous Body by Jake series attests that weight training builds more than strong muscles in youth. Mastery in one area such as strength training quickly translates into self-esteem and competence in other areas of a teen's life. "I want you to build the most impressive physique that you thought possible," Steinfeld advises teenagers in his book *Get Strong*, "but I also want you to build an impressive future."

dieting tips to solutions for inactive families. Each check-in is designed to keep you motivated and on track.

Most of the exercises presented are suitable for all ages. Do note, however, that the more challenging exercises are labeled as such and should only be attempted when you are ready. Knee, back, or shoulder problems can appear at any age, so wherever possible I have included modifications. Instructions will tell you the goal of each exercise, the breathing pattern, and what key muscles are being worked. Read the instructions thoroughly before attempting an exercise.

The exercises are presented in a way that facilitates a smooth transition on or off the ball and into the next move, so try and follow the order as much as possible. The sequence is also designed to utilize muscles in order: warming them up and preparing them for the next exercise. The watchpoints should be read closely and followed for your own safety and enjoyment. People who are recovering from an injury may need to begin rehabilitation on a stable surface instead of a ball. See your medical practitioner to make sure these exercises are for you.

Recently I found the dictionary definition of *functional* scribbled among the diagrams of the first exercises Liuda and I did together. *Functional* is defined as "contributing to the development or maintenance of a larger whole," implying a sense of cooperation. Cooperation is in fact exactly what we are trying to achieve in *Strength Training on the Ball.*

In both everyday situations such as placing a can of food in a cupboard and in moments of athletic vigor such as slamming a hockey puck while withstanding a body check, the body works as a unit. The premise of my book is that we should be training the body to address this fact. My deepest hope is that you will fully embrace this safe and functional approach to strength training and in a short time delight in its benefits.

1

The Ball and
The Method

*The balls are dynamic
playmates on which we
cannot intellectualize about
our mobility.*
—Somatic educator
Ninoska Gómez

*I like using the ball because
it is fun.*
—From *Kids on the Ball*

Aquilino's Story

It is a sparkling bright October day when I board the northbound train at Florence. The Bologna stop comes quickly. Outside the train window I see only a hint of fall color, nothing compared to the hard yellows and reds I left in Canada two days ago. Udine is the final stop, five hours by train from Florence, in the far northeast corner of Italy, almost at the Slovenian border. This is my destination.

In a brief stop at Treviso, the carriage empties and my excitement builds. This is for me a pilgrimage of sorts. The man who I have come to see on this warm autumn day is Aquilino Cosani. Described by some as an Italian plastics manufacturer, by others as a toy maker, he is the man who created the process in which large colorful balls could be molded, cooled, and filled with air. He is the inventor of the first exercise ball.

The sun-drenched landscape rushes by as the train moves northward. The small village of Osoppo, near Udine, is the location of the Cosani factory. There is another toy manufacturer in the same area called Trudi, which makes teddy bears and other animals so soft and threadbare they appear as if their fur has already been loved off them. I recognize a Trudi cat with broad padded feet peeking out of one of the elegant bags of an Italian grandmother who disembarked at Treviso and wonder again about Mr. Cosani: What kind of toys, if any, will I find at the end of this journey?

From his son I know this. Aquilino Cosani was born in 1924, the first of eight brothers born in Romania to Italian parents. His father relocated to Romania in the early 1920s looking for work as a housebuilder to feed his growing family. Eventually the family returned to Italy and Aquilino studied to become an engineer. Then he traveled to Milan and worked in the Pirelli factory—a factory where they created overshoes, tires, and other products in rubber. He absorbed as much as he could and thought long and hard about how rubber manufacturing could be improved upon. In 1948 he returned to the village of Osoppo and started, with only the help of a friend, to make rubber Pinocchios and animal toys in the basement of his house. Little by little his Pinocchios and duckies multiplied and in 1963 he needed to move his operations to the industrial outskirts of the town as he began to export to other parts of Europe. By this time his line had expanded to include beach balls.

I meet Mr. Cosani outside the white and blue factory, behind which the foothills of the Alps spread dramatically. Gone are all my stereotypes of Pinocchio's shabby, long-haired, toy-maker father clad in overalls and an apron. Mr. Aquilino Cosani, a very distinguished man in his late seventies, is dressed in a suit and tie. Still very active in the business, he meets for a simple lunch every day with his sons. Nevio Cosani, his oldest son, is responsible for marketing and accounting for a factory that today offers over 150 products. He moves us into an impressive showroom flaunting balls of all sizes and colors and begins to translate for us. I am delighted to find out that Mr. Cosani speaks French. When Nevio leaves us alone for a few minutes, unburdened by wooden translations, Mr. Cosani becomes much less formal as we converse in French. His eyes twinkle as he remembers his surprise—no, forty years ago he had no idea what an adult would do with a ball.

I know the outline of the ball's history from physical therapist and ball pioneer Joanne Posner-Mayer's book *Swiss Ball Applications for Orthopedic and Sport Medicine*. Posner-Mayer, a graduate of the University of Colorado's School of Physical Therapy, had the opportunity in the 1970s to practice for seven years with influential and progressive therapists in Switzerland, including the Czech physiotherapist Frau Maria Kucera and therapists trained by Dr. Susanne Klein-Vogelbach. Dr. Klein-Vogelbach was the first to use balls with adults with orthopedic and postural problems.

The story of using a ball for therapy probably begins in the late 1950s, when the Swiss pediatrician Dr. Elsbeth Köng went to England to learn the Bobath Method of neuromuscular reeducation. Köng invited Mary Quinton, an English physiotherapist, to work with her in Switzerland; together they developed programs using beach balls to work with neurologically impaired children and babies. Klein-Vogelbach was then introduced to the balls by a colleague who had attended a Mary Quinton class on the Bobath Method, and she went on to pioneer ball exercises, theory, and clinical applications of the ball for adults.

According to Mr. Cosani, sometime around 1963, Dr. Susanne Klein-Vogelbach approached one of his distributors in Switzerland with an unusual request. Could the Italian toy maker create a ball large and sturdy enough so that adult patients recovering from serious back operations could use it safely? Cosani agreed and the rest is history.

Who would have guessed? A ball had significantly transformed Mr. Cosani's life just as it had mine. I ruminate on this for a second and then ask: "Do you remember how many adult balls were originally made?"

He pauses for a moment. He believes somewhere between one hundred and two hundred balls were first manufactured and sent off to Switzerland. What concerned him was the consistency of the ball. In the beginning he had started with a pungent rubber latex from Asia; he then moved to plastic, which was more elastic. Finally he switched to a nontoxic, latex free, easy-to-clean vinyl.

"I see," I nod. "You fulfilled the request. But did you have an idea what this shipment would mean, that it would be the beginning of something much bigger?"

"No," he responds in French with one firm shake of the head. "I did not."

After I take my leave of the gracious Aquilino Cosani, Nevio leads me on a tour of the ball factory. I meet the other son, Paolo, the technical director, who is responsible for the manufacturing of the balls. I am shown the two-piece cast-iron shell where the liquid raw material is poured and rotated but am not allowed to take a photograph of it. Anyone can throw PVC dust together with chemicals and oils, but it is the exact formula of this, as well as the uniqueness of the machines, that gives the Italian balls their special, burst-resistant texture and pleasant vanilla scent. I run my fingers across the soft, still warm, ear of a Rody Horse ball as it comes out of its mold. A Rody is really a hopping ball that allows a young child the benefits of bouncing with stability. Further along, I come upon an unusual peanut-shaped ball called a Physio Roll cooling on a rack.

"Do you know what I heard today?" Nevio asks, as we stand over the two balls in one. He shows me an e-mail from a veterinarian who uses a 45-centimeter Physio Roll, with its wide base of support, to help dogs regain muscle mass after surgery or trauma. I smile widely at the idea of this: the ball moving from kids to adults to animals. The era of the ball has truly arrived.

The Pilates Method: Over Ninety Years Old and Growing Strong

Truth will prevail and that is why I know my teachings will reach the masses and finally be adopted as universal.
—Joseph H. Pilates

The day after I visited the Cosani factory, I was invited to Studio Pilates Quaranta, Udine's first Pilates studio. Northeast Italy's second largest city, Udine has an exquisite and blissfully tourist-free medieval square. Paola del Fabbro, a former high school physical education teacher who has recently given up her post to devote herself full time to her Pilates studio, whisked me past the square, pointing out its Venetian influences, before continuing to her studio. "We are still building, I'm afraid," she murmured in almost perfect English. "I must have an urgent word with the builder. We must open by Monday."

We parked on a quiet street and I followed Paola upstairs. One worker was sawing while the other was laying the wooden beams of the floor. As I stepped into the room I caught my breath: at once I saw how perfect the studio will be. The windows were full length and the room had that spacious, exclusive yet friendly, serene feeling that so many of the best Pilates studios have.

Paola took me upstairs to her apartment, directly above the studio, to show me the Pilates equipment she had stored there. When she left me to have a final word with the builders, I surveyed her beautiful flat. All was still. I watched a ray of sunlight from the window streak across the solid-oak-framed Pilates Reformer onto the upholstered headrest.

What would Joseph Hubertus Pilates have made of studios in his name not only opening all over North America but also in the Far East, Australia, South Africa, South America, and of course Europe? Exquisitely crafted leather barrels and pricey chrome- or oak-framed Reformers with leather straps and thick springs are now available around the world; cheaper versions of these as well as the Pilates Chair, Cadillac, and Trapezuis are popping up on infomercials for home use.

Born in 1880 near Dusseldorf, Germany, Joseph Pilates had been a sickly boy; his athletic feats were his personal quest to solve his own health problems. When World War I broke out he had been living in England instructing detectives on self-defense and working as a circus performer and boxer. Because of his nationality he was interned in Lancashire and later on the Isle of Man. Today the folklore on "Uncle Joe" has created its own momentum and anecdotes; how he became a nurse in the camp and treated inmates, some recovering from horrendous war injuries, using ropes, pulleys, and bedsprings, anything he could get his hands on. Not to mention the fact that the influenza epidemic of 1918 was raging, yet not a single internee held with Joseph Pilates was affected. Apparently everyone in the camp, guards and prisoners, was doing his exercises.

He was ahead of his time when he brought his ideas on body conditioning and rehabilitation to the New World. Joseph Pilates immigrated to New York in the late 1920s and with his wife, Clara, a nurse he met on the boat to America, opened a studio on Eighth Avenue. In the 1930s and 1940s, choreographers and dancers such as Martha Graham, George Balanchine, and Jerome Robbins sought him out and then fully embraced his method. Today, everywhere from the local Y to the neighborhood church or community center offers a class in Pilates. Group mat classes, which have popularized Pilates, are a relatively new phenomenon in the last few years. The majority of Pilates students still practice Pilates in a studio. They work individually with a trainer in programs designed for the student. Others learn the method from the many books or tapes that have appeared in fitness sections of bookstores and department stores.

Believe it or not, when I began studying Pilates in 1997 there was only one book available on the Pilates Method—Philip Friedman and Gail Eisen's *The Pilates Method of Physical and Mental Conditioning* published in 1980. Dedicated to Joseph and Clara Pilates, and the doyenne of the Pilates Method, Romana Kryzanowska, the authors studied in the Pilates Studio in New York, wrote the book, and appeared in the photos. By the time I began to study

The Evolution of the Pilates Method

When Joseph Pilates died in 1967, he left no single teacher or protégé to carry on with this work. His wife, Clara, continued to operate the studio and Romana Kryzanowska became the director. Romana and a handful of other Pilates students passed down from teacher to teacher different perspectives on the work. Each of these first-generation teachers, inspired by their dance and other backgrounds, added their own important innovations and modifications to the program. Some specialized in a more functional approach to Pilates, using Pilates to correct faulty alignment and imbalances in the body. Others focused on the exercises as an art form—a dance on mats—the goal being to perfect the movements as you increased their difficulty.

The legacy that has been left by the first-generation teachers and their students is a system of stretching and strengthening exercises designed to repattern the body and to use the mind to educate (or reeducate) the body via the nervous system. Whether we swing a golf club or pick up a child, nerves carry signals from the mind to the muscles, telling the muscles why and how to contract. Pilates practitioners use isolated movements to reeducate the body, teaching the nervous system to recruit the weak areas, not just the strong ones. This is why Pilates exercises are often done at low levels of intensity. We focus on quality of movement, not quantity, to make sure the body is aligned properly and the correct muscles are working. Pilates can be done at high levels of intensity, but only when the stabilizers, or core muscles, are strong and the nervous system is working correctly.

11

Pilates the book was out of print and impossible to get. I borrowed a ragged copy from one of the trainees in my group and studied it long into the night, as it had to be returned the next day to its owner who was going back to the States. I felt a bit like the Soviet dissident intellectuals I had heard about from my friend Liuda who, cut off from certain literature and political tracts, circulated among themselves *samizdat*, illegal copies of forbidden literature, often staying up all night to read a tract before passing it on.

Joseph Pilates wrote his own books, the most well-known being *Return to Life Through Contrology*, written in 1945 but only widely available in the late 1990s when it was reprinted by Judd Robbins and Lin Van Heuit-Robbins. Dedicated to Pilates' wife, Clara, it is a slender book, written with William J. Miller. It highlights Pilates' philosophy and his exercise system, which he called Contrology. He described his system as a "complete coordination of body, mind and spirit." At the time he must have had his disbelievers, but today the method has been around too long to be a passing fancy.

Pilates is very well supported by people in conventional and alternative health and movement fields. Many physical therapists, chiropractors, osteopaths, and other rehabilitation workers are using the method for orthopedic and geriatric patients, neurologic rehabilitation, and pain relief. Suddenly the demand for Pilates is outstripping the availability of teachers—some Pilates certification programs in North America and in the United Kingdom find themselves fully booked up to a year in advance.

Why Pilates-Based Ballwork?

I began integrating balls into my group mat classes in 1998 because I was concerned that my group students were not receiving weight-bearing, resistance, and balance training from the ordinary matwork. As any student of a Pilates mat class can attest, most if not all of the hour is experienced down on the mat, many exercises performed in a supine, or lying on the back, position. Remaining as faithful as possible to my Pilates training and experience, I went one by one through all the mat and apparatus-based exercises to see which exercises could be adapted to the ball. Though the ball works differently on the body than a piece of Pilates apparatus does, the ball has some definite advantages, not the least being that the ball allows a student to get off the mat and into functional, three-dimensional movement. Working with small and large balls changes the body's relationship to gravity, enhances stretching and lengthening, and uniquely challenges the nervous and musculoskeletal systems, providing an opportunity for students to also train for better balance in the process. Functional movement explorations and balance challenges prepare students for more efficiently and safely executing tasks in their sports activities and everyday lives.

Moreover, the ball is the perfect partner in a Pilates approach to strength training. First, the body is worked through multiple planes. The limbs of the body are meant to twist and rotate, swivel inward and outward, not to move only in one plane as is simulated on traditional weight machines. Working the limbs at various angles, on diagonals, across the body, and in circles forces more individual muscles into play and stimulates many more muscles and joints.

In addition to working the limbs through a full range of motion, strength training on the ball utilizes the body as a unit. Working on the ball, deep postural muscles and other stabilizers work along with larger muscles. A greater range of muscle fibers is engaged, the muscles contracting and relaxing as necessary, and correct sequencing and cooperation between the muscles is encouraged. This is functional strength training at its very best, promising great results for beginners, those recovering from injuries, and seasoned athletes.

The intersection of the ball with my life was an accident. I had no idea that this partnership between the ball and the Pilates Method would have such far-reaching consequences for me personally and professionally. I was reaching toward an impulse—a need to give my group mat students balance-training, weight-bearing, and resistance experiences and to see if we could adapt some of the equipment-based exercises to the ball. Today the ball has a solid place in the Pilates repertoire; many Pilates teachers and personal trainers are using balls instead of the expensive equipment and devising their own applications.

Check-In: Getting Started

In the next chapter we will explore the mechanics of movement and how breath influences movement. But what if you are not able to begin a movement program at all? This is much more common than you might think.

Eric Maisel is a psychotherapist who has inspired many writers, musicians, and visual artists to work through disabling emotional blocks and embark on new ventures. I pass on his words here, as I think the stakes are no higher for a frustrated artist than they are for a menopausal women with a family history of osteoporosis who knows she must take up strength training yet simply does not know how to begin. "Every day you will need to restart," advises Maisel, adding: "How can you restart undramatically and untraumatically the next million times?"

Beginning a fitness program "undramatically" and "untraumatically" may mean seriously looking inside yourself to see what voices you are carrying from

advantages of using the ball for strength training

- Targets deep as well as superficial muscles
- Adds resistance and weight bearing to mat exercises
- Works the body as a unit more functionally than a stable bench
- Manipulates angle of effort and works through full range of motion and multiple planes
- Trains the muscles to work together, engaging more muscle fibers and encouraging correct sequencing
- Creates higher demand on motor system and nervous system
- Induces relaxation and fun

Belligerently commit to starting.
—Eric Maisel, Ph.D.,
Fearless Creating

13

the past. You need to calm the censoring voice inside that tells you that what you are about to do is silly, that you are too old, too fat, too skinny, that you have no time, that you will fail at strength training. This voice blocks your good intentions as it makes you believe it is simply trying to take care of you, a leftover from the days when others used negative phrases to protect you from harm.

Next, seriously evaluate your lifestyle and exercise habits. Perhaps you absolutely need a class or a workout partner to stay motivated. What about variety—are you doing the same thing over and over? Do you need to hire a personal trainer to help set you up on a program, show you some new moves, and help you find the balance between weight-bearing and aerobic exercise? Perhaps not starting is about your own health or previous injury concerns. Make an appointment with a physical therapist or other health professional to see if you are ready to start. If you are menopausal, discuss osteoporosis with your doctor and inquire about a bone-density test. If there are other reasons why you cannot begin, talk to a friend or a therapist about what is blocking you from taking charge of your health.

We are the "block"
we perceive.
—Julia Cameron,
The Artist's Way

Julia Cameron, an author who has helped countless would-be creators and others to take charge of their lives, warns about the "creative U-turn," the point when people abandon their endeavors and return to what was. When she teaches the Artist's Way seminar, she requires her students to make a contract with themselves, which they sign and date, committing to the work of the course as well as to "excellent self-care, adequate sleep, diet, exercise and pampering." What a terrific strategy: because for some, beginning is easy—it's staying committed that is extremely challenging.

Make a contract today that you will stay committed to your health. Sign and date this promise to keep your bones strong and your body moving. Commit to paper what changes you would like to make to improve your health. Note long-term and short-term goals. Be as specific as possible. Your long-term goals may include eliminating stress, smoking, and the overuse of alcohol and caffeine. Your short-term goal may be to walk a certain distance every week, starting today. Or to visit a nearby gym, inspect its weight room, and note if its class schedule would work for you.

Track your progress. What you are now doing for exercise, if anything? Does your list include a balance between strength training, aerobic activities, and stretching? Next, jot down a strategy that will help alleviate your fears right now. Finally, do something practical. Purchase two pairs of free weights (dumbbells) and put them where you can see them. I would suggest a pair of 1- or 2-pound weights and, depending on your fitness level, 3- or 5-pound weights to begin with. Blow up the ball and see that in fact only a corner of a room is necessary to get started—you don't need a home gym. If a year's membership at a gym is too daunting, then take the booklet of ten passes or a three-month membership. Or sign up for a ten-week movement class; there are usually no refunds and you will be forced to give it a try to get your money's worth.

Set realistic goals and keep a journal of what you do each week. Note obstacles. If you have to skip a few workouts, don't let guilt build up to be another block in your path or a hurdle in your commitment. Get back on schedule immediately and forget the past. Avoid all-or-nothing thinking. Just twenty minutes a day can make a real difference.

Embarking on a strength-training program can change your life but it can also save your life. Is there anything more important than your health?

2
Breathing
and Releasing

Maria's Story: Freeing the Rib Cage

The injury was the result of performing a back somersault into a shallow part of a lagoon on the rugged south coast of South Africa. Maria had fractured a vertebra that could only be mended by a complicated and invasive surgery. Her doctor did not prepare her for the fact that after the operation she would be placed first back downward and then stomach downward into a bath of soft plaster of paris so that a customized back brace could be cast for her. The brace, which was meant to keep her back immobile while her bones knitted, had to be worn day and night. The spinal fusion occurred seventeen years ago, but what Maria most remembers of the weeks that followed the operation was that she could not get a full breath.

Maria is an asthma sufferer. When she was ten, a South African specialist in asthma explained to her how related the diaphragm is to other body structures. He taught her to use the inhalation to fill her whole chest cavity as deeply and widely as possible by expanding her ribs as far as they would go. After this she had to exhale as hard as she could through her mouth. Joseph Pilates himself was asthmatic and he experimented with breath. He spoke of "squeezing every atom of pure air from your lungs": the importance of a full exhalation and a full inhalation.

The brace was put on a few days after the operation. It felt like second skin except that this skin was rock hard and inflexible. Maria could not expand her rib cage and utilize the key muscles in the breathing process—the intercostal (rib cage) and the accessory muscles of the back—as she had been taught. Instead the body cast forced her to breathe shallowly in the upper part of her chest. She was suffocating and had to be administered tranquilizers to relax.

Over the months that she had to endure the brace Maria had one recurring dream. She dreamed of a time when she was a child and how, while inhaling in front of an open window, she would fling both arms wide as if welcoming a lost relative before exhaling with as much force as she could muster.

The Three-Dimensional Breath

When you breathe this is what happens. The windpipe (the trachea) takes the air into the bronchia, which branch into millions of tiny air sacs to convey the air into the lungs. Oxygen is drawn into the blood through these air sacs and is carried by the red blood cells until it reaches the capillaries. The oxygen is then absorbed by the tissues of the body and exchanged for carbon dioxide. Carbon dioxide, one of the waste products of the body, takes the reverse route from the tissues and working muscles back through the veins to be exhaled on the out breath from the body.

The diaphragm, a dome-shaped muscle between the chest and the abdominals, is the principal breathing muscle. It is designed to work like a pump: on the in breath it contracts and, because of differing pressure outside and inside the body, air is drawn inside. On the out breath the diaphragm relaxes and the dome rises, discharging used air. If unrestricted, the diaphragm not only moves up and down but also billows outward.

In the Pilates approach we try to guide the breath not into the upper chest but into the lower rib cage. This is called back breathing. Back breathing utilizes the full spectrum of breathing muscles as well as the deep transversus abdominal and oblique muscles that contract the abdominal area. Pilates breathing is often called "lateral breathing" because the aim is to expand the rib cage sideways on the inhalation.

As we attempt three-dimensional breathing we do not want to restrict the natural ballooning of the belly; we want the abdominals to gently rise and fall with breath. Chronic tight contraction of the abdominals pulls down on the lower ribs and interferes with the pumplike downward motion of the diaphragm. So in daily life we do not want a chronic tight contraction of the abdominals. However, when we initiate a movement, whether it's lifting a weight (think of taking a heavy bag of groceries from the back of your car) or extending the spine to place an object on a high shelf we need to make sure

17

that the deep abdominals are fully engaged to protect the low back. In a Pilates approach we use the breath—primarily the exhalation—to engage the deep abdominals, gently drawing the navel inward before each and every movement. This connection is called the navel-to-spine connection. It is a fundamental concept that will be discussed further in the next chapter and throughout the book.

In Pilates we use the breath not only to better oxygenate the blood but to create a strong abdominal-pelvic core. We also use the breath to release specific muscles that are overworking and need to let go. We will see in the next chapter how the deep postural muscles support the spine and stabilize the joints. However, more often than not it's the outer layer of muscles that is guilty of overworking, taking over tasks for which they are not designed.

Supplying Oxygen to the Muscles

exercise helps the body improve its ability to transport and use oxygen, and correct breathing nurtures the body and releases toxins. We use more oxygen during exercise than we do when we are at rest. To get the oxygen necessary in a more vigorous workout, we need to take in a greater quantity of air. Make sure the area where you exercise is well-ventilated.

Air is drawn in through the nose. Oxygen is taken to the working muscles by the hemoglobin in the blood. In the thin-walled capillaries, oxygen is exchanged for carbon dioxide and exhaled by the body.

Training the cardiovascular system makes the heart recover quicker from rigorous exertion. Athletes test this by taking their pulse levels during and after a workout. Athletes who train at high altitudes have more hemoglobin than others because their bodies have adapted to the lower concentration of available oxygen. Generally, people who are in good physical condition have more hemoglobin and the ability to get a greater amount of oxygen to their muscles in a shorter period of time.

In a Pilates workout we are mindful as to how we breathe because correct breathing not only supplies oxygen to the working muscles but helps to create a strong core by activating the deep abdominal muscles. Of primary importance is removing the effort from breathing. Especially do not force the inhalation, as this may cause lightheadedness. On the out breath—a purposeful breath through the mouth—unused gases stored in the body are expelled. The goal is natural breathing. Above all, do not hold your breath.

Focused breathing can help you drop your shoulders, create release in the large superficial muscles of the torso and legs, and help the body reeducate itself so that the postural and breathing muscles work together to stabilize your core.

Efficient breathing is essential for the survival of man and beast, whether the breath is used to pour energy and force into the skeletal muscles or to relax the body. In his wise and beautifully written book *Yoga and the Quest for the True Self*, Stephen Cope writes about the breath as being a "switching station" between the physical body and energy body. Many of us do not breathe properly and in fact only use a fraction of our lung capacity. Cope reminds us that full diaphragmatic breathing stimulates the alpha waves associated with relaxation, whereas chest breathing has a negative impact on the physical body and the nervous system and causes tension to accumulate in the jaw, the mouth, and between the shoulder blades. When the lungs and diaphragm are not restricted, writes Cope, we have full access to our internal emotional experience.

The ball is an excellent tool to help you approach relaxation and release. "Moving on the balls helps us massage our internal organs and get direct experience of the content-container relationship between the organs and skeletal-muscular structure," Ninoska Gómez, Ph.D., writes of her Somarhythms ballwork. In addition to placing the body in different relationships to gravity, small and large balls can help you physically see and feel the breath being channeled into different parts of the body.

Rest As You Go: An Italian Story

Tonight's class at the fitness center Ceron in Udine, Italy, is for women only. I watch a group of twenty-five graceful, middle-aged, Italian women select a mat, a large ball, and two small balls—one with a smooth surface, the other, a knobby ball.

I am here only to observe and the first indication that I am in for something different is the music: a mix between muted operatic and New Age. Enrico Ceron adjusts the volume. On his head is a microphone set used by many aerobic teachers around the world, but this is no ordinary class. After a warm-up he leads the women into a series of upper- and lower-body strength moves using smooth baby-blue 9-inch balls. My favorite are a series of sitting-on-the-ball exercises for the abdominals and legs.

Then, when their muscles are straining, Enrico has the women switch to the small knobby-surfaced balls. The knobby balls have small spikes used to promote blood circulation and get at tight muscles. His voice softens and the women slowly roll and press the spiky balls around their heads and necks and down their limbs, enhancing sensations and stimulating acupressure points. Many of the women's eyes are closed. The release in their bodies is visible.

After more strengthening exercises, Ceron's class ends with an unexpected twist. He dims the lights and switches to honey-sweet flute music. The women, accustomed to this finish, get into position. One woman lies on her belly on the mat while a classmate unhurriedly rolls the large ball from head to toe over the back surface of her partner's body. She draws one hand over the other, dexterously, as if stroking an ancient instrument and not an air-filled ball. Then the woman begins making tiny hypnotic ball-taps, moving up and down, left and right, and drawing circles and figure 8s on the back of the prone body. As I watch, release traces a slow path down my spine and into my belly.

The women change positions. My notebook is open but I have forgotten to take a single note. I think to myself: All this time I've taught ball classes and yet I've never seen anything like this. Afterward I find one woman who speaks English. "Do you come to this class often?" I ask a dark-eyed, full-bodied Venus before she exits.

"As often as I can," she says with a smile, her eyes soft with repose.

"Relaxation is not negation, it is not passivity," attests Mabel E. Todd, author of the classic *The Thinking Body*. She reminds us that in all living cells and systems, nature provides two phrases of bodily rhythm: work and rest. One balances the other. Why push mercilessly through a nonstop workout when utilizing a "rest and activity rhythm" would conserve energy and create pleasure in movement?

Just settling on the mat may be challenging for a person who is overextended and used to being on the run or always surrounded by others. You meet yourself on the mat, alone, with no distraction, and you might not like what you see. Don't judge your initial reactions: the more you become accustomed to relaxing, the easier it will become.

A relaxation position or "breather" creates the mind space needed to go quiet and listen to your body. In a Pilates-based workout these relaxation positions are built into the session. We momentarily pause before each exercise, scan the body, and ensure that we're in good alignment. This is not an opportunity to let everything go and sprawl on your mat. In the words of Mabel Todd: "Take hold of your bones softly but do not let go of them."

The Breathing Exercises

The breath is a powerful force and an important aid in strength training. The breathing patterns that accompany each exercise in this book are not written in stone and should be adjusted to meet the needs of each student. The general rule is to use the inhalation to prepare the body and mentally to check the postural alignment. This means for some students to use the inhalation to release the shoulder blades away from the ears or to lengthen the spine while either lying on the mat or sitting up on the ball. Sometimes the inhalation is used to ensure that the buttocks, forehead, mouth, jaw, and back of the neck are released and that the fingertips are not unconsciously clutching the side of the mat. The exhalation is often used to engage the deep abdominals and other core muscles as you move into the exertion phase of the exercise. Many Pilates exercises require more than one movement; so you will often inhale in the middle of an exercise and use the exhalation to again ensure the core muscles are engaged as you complete the movement. In some cases the exhalation is used to return the body to a relaxing position back on the mat or the ball. The goal is natural breathing, not forced breathing. Above all, do not hold your breath.

In the Pilates approach to the breath we inhale through the nose and exhale through the mouth with slightly pursed lips. Some Pilates practitioners teach that a controlled exhalation through pursed lips facilitates the deep contraction of the transversus abdominis as well as the sphincter muscles of the pelvic floor. It is important, however, not to force the exhalation. Imagine steadily blowing a flickering candle; do not blow it out. Some students, especially in the beginning, find the breathing very challenging. If you try too hard you may become dizzy or light-headed. Try to discover the bottom of the exhalation—the moment of calm before the next in-breath. Joseph Pilates used a device like a pinwheel to help students physically see the little wheel spin as a result of their long, relaxing exhale.

Some exercises call for percussive breathing: three to five staccato "blows" and three to five staccato "sniffs." This unique approach warms the body and stimulates the diaphragm.

As you work through the exercises in this book you will see that there is a choreographed breathing pattern to accompany each exercise. The breathing patterns help one movement blend into the next. A sense of flow is important when doing strength training with lighter-than-usual weights. We do not rest between sets when we are building endurance and functional strength. With precision and good alignment we weave one move into the next, marrying the breath with the movement.

Ball Breathing

I want to begin by reminding you that the goal of Pilates breathing is not to breathe into the belly. Pilates practitioners do not recommend belly breathing while performing exercises because a loose belly relaxes the abdominal muscles, creating instability in the low back and pelvis. Instead the aim is to engage the deep abdominals and other core muscles on the exhalation and, if possible, to keep these supporting muscles engaged while you expand your rib cage on the inhalation.

Belly breathing, movement 1, however, is excellent for encouraging relaxation. Sometimes I begin my classes with belly breathing to encourage release and to remind my students what we are *not* trying to achieve. Drape your hands across your belly to feel it balloon upward as you inhale. In movements 2 and 3 we begin to practice the Pilates back breathing, sometimes called lateral breathing; here the emphasis is on sending the breath into the rib cage, not the belly. Wrap your hands around the rib cage in movement 2 and add a gentle resistance. In movement 3, side breathing, notice how the ball provides a gentle resistance against the side of the rib cage, increasing your sensory awareness. Can you feel the upper rib cage, the part toward the ceiling, expand on your inhalation? Side breathing is for anyone who for whatever reason is not comfortable lying on the back. Remember to inhale through the nose and exhale through the mouth with slightly pursed lips.

Purpose Movement 1 is for relaxation. Movements 2 and 3 practice the lateral breathing used for most Pilates-based work.

Watchpoints • Keep the body relaxed to experience the breath move through the body. • Think of breathing into the lower back of the lungs, not the front of the chest. • Inhale through the nose and exhale through the mouth.

starting position

Lie on your back with your legs suspended up on the ball. Rest your hands on your belly. If desired, close your eyes.

movement 1: belly breathing

1. Inhale through the nose for four counts to expand the belly **(fig. 2.1)**.
2. Exhale through slightly pursed lips for four or five counts to release. Find your full exhale.
3. Take five breaths, slow and deep, in this manner.

movement 2: back breathing

1. Wrap your hands around your ribs with the fingers around the front and side and the thumbs on the back **(fig. 2.2)**. Apply slight resistance. Inhale for four or five counts, feeling your rib cage expand into your fingers.
2. Exhale through slightly pursed lips for five counts to release. On the exhalation, practice gently drawing the navel in toward the spine.
3. Take five breaths in this manner, practicing widening the rib cage into your fingers.

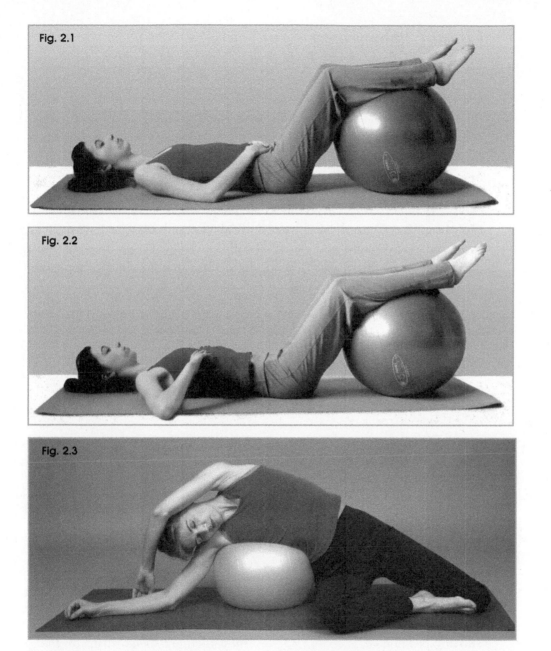

Fig. 2.1

Fig. 2.2

Fig. 2.3

movement 3: side breathing

1. Sit with your right side beside your ball. Bend the right knee in front and curl the left foot behind you. Shift your weight onto the right side and allow the right side of the body to release over the ball, left arm relaxing overhead. Rest your head on your right shoulder **(fig. 2.3)**.

2. Inhale through the nose to expand the rib cage.
3. Exhale through slightly pursed lips to release. On the exhalation, practice gently drawing the navel inward.
4. Take five more breaths in this manner, then repeat on the other side.

23

Chest Opener with Arm Circles

Chest Openers can be done on the mat or on a small (9-inch) underinflated ball. Try the exercises on the mat first and use the inhalation to open up any restricted parts of the body. The small ball, positioned between the bottom of the shoulder blades, causes the muscles of the upper back to release so once you remove the ball the spine and neck are lengthened. To come out of this movement, place your hands behind your head and lift the head. Then roll to one side off the small ball, pulling your knees to your chest.

Purpose To release the spine, abdominals, back of neck, and shoulders.

Watchpoints • Control the rib cage; don't allow your back to arch off the mat as you move your arms. • In the small-ball version, make sure that the neck is safe. • Use a cushion under the head if necessary. • Be sure that long hair does not get stuck under the ball.

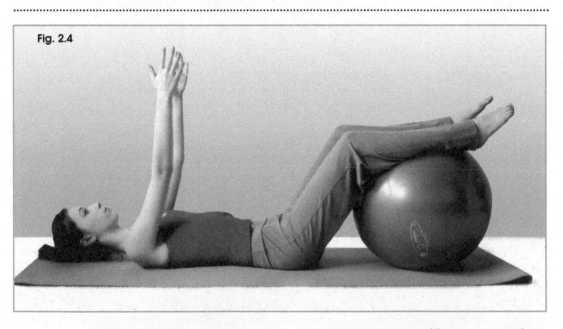

Fig. 2.4

starting position

Lie on your back with your knees bent, your lower legs resting on the ball. Feet should be hip-distance apart and parallel, in line with your knees; knees are in line with your hips. Fingers are stretched down by the thighs, with your palms facing the body.

movement 1: soldier arms on the mat

1. Raise both arms above the shoulders, hands shoulder-distance apart. The palms face each other **(fig. 2.4)**.
2. On the exhalation lower your left arm toward your left ear and your right arm toward the mat **(fig. 2.5)**.

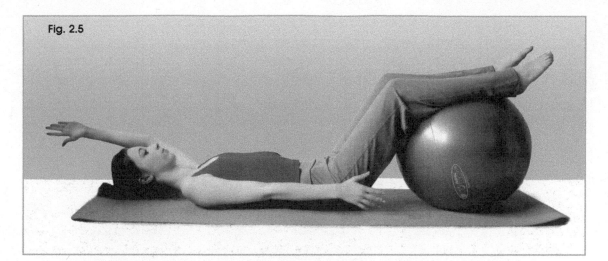

Fig. 2.5

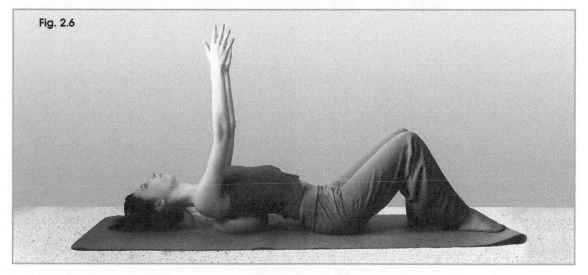

Fig. 2.6

3. Inhale to lift both arms above the shoulders, shoulder-distance apart, palms facing each other.

4. Exhale to lower your right arm toward your right ear and your left arm toward the mat.

5. Repeat three to five times on each side.

movement 2: soldier arms on small ball

1. Roll to one side and slip the small ball between the bottom of your shoulder blades. Roll back onto the ball. Clasp your hands behind your head and slowly lower the head to a safe position. Knees are bent, feet are parallel and in line with the knees. Start with both arms extended above your shoulders, hands shoulder-distance apart and palms facing each other **(fig. 2.6)**.

25

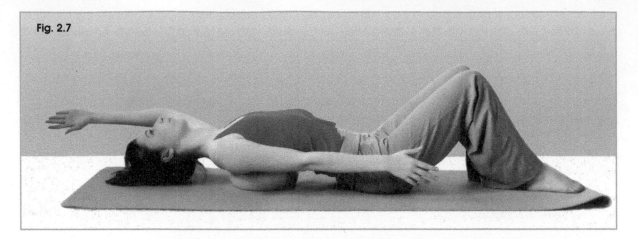

Fig. 2.7

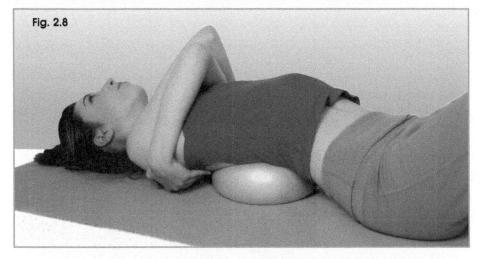

Fig. 2.8

2. On the exhalation lower the left arm toward your left ear and your right arm toward the mat **(fig. 2.7)**.

3. Inhale to lift both arms above the shoulders, shoulder-distance apart, palms facing each other.

4. Exhale to lower your right arm toward your right ear and your left arm to the mat.

5. Repeat three to five times on each side.

movement 3: body hugs on the small ball

1. Wrap your arms around your upper body, reaching for the shoulder blades **(fig. 2.8)**. On the inhalation, give yourself a gentle hug. On the exhalation, open the arms to the side.

2. Wrap the other arm on top and repeat.

Breathing and The Hundred

Movement 1 in this next series is adapted from a beginner-level exercise on the Cadillac, one of the specialized pieces of equipment that Joseph Pilates developed. Don't rush the action—this exercise is usually performed on an apparatus whose springs automatically slow you down. As you coordinate your breath with the movement, note that you are moving all four ball-and-socket joints at once—the two hip joints and the two shoulder joints. The buttocks will work as you slowly lift your pelvis in the air in time with the arm movement, but it's the deep abdominal connection that controls the "unrolling" motion of the spine. Movement 2, the hundred, is a great mat exercise but is underused by Pilates teachers as the fantastic breathing exercise it is. The hundred gets the blood circulating and warms the body with its percussive breathing. Make sure you're moving the arms directly from the shoulder joint, not from your wrists or elbows. For now keep your head down on the mat and sink the navel in toward the spine on the exhalation.

Purpose To coordinate breath with movement.

Watchpoints • In movement 2, the hundred, make sure the entire arm moves from the socket and not from the wrist or elbow. • Keep elbows soft, not hyperextended. • Don't let the torso move as you pump the arms, and keep the shoulders down. Inhale through the nose and exhale through the mouth with slightly pursed lips.

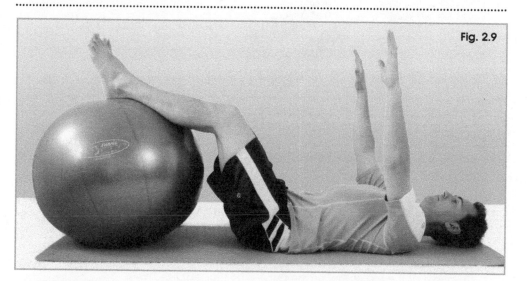

Fig. 2.9

starting position

Suspend your legs on the ball. Keep the legs in good alignment: feet in line with the ankles, ankles in line with the knees.

movement 1: breathing

1. Lift your arms in the air directly above the shoulders **(fig. 2.9)**. Inhale to prepare.

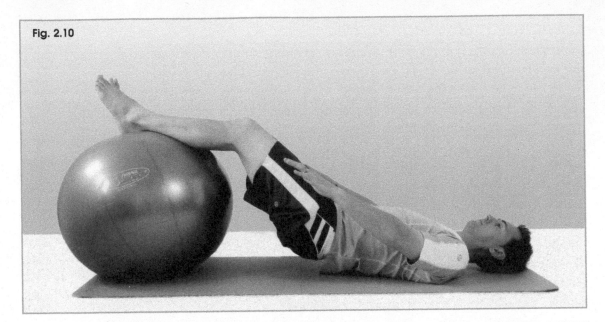

Fig. 2.10

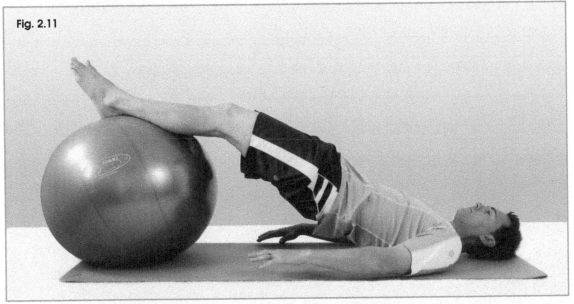

Fig. 2.11

2. Exhale to drop the navel and lengthen the tailbone away from the pelvis. Then curl the pelvis up at the same time as the arms press slowly and simultaneously downward **(fig. 2.10)**.

3. Inhale at the top of the movement. Arms are hovering beside you just off the mat **(fig. 2.11)**.

4. Exhale and roll the pelvis downward, letting the deep abdominal connection control your movement. Your arms slowly return to above the shoulders **(fig. 2.12)**.

5. Repeat five times.

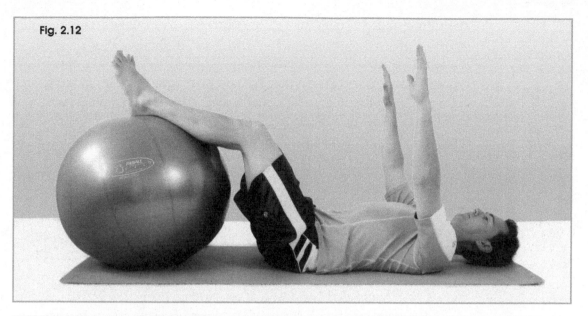

Fig. 2.12

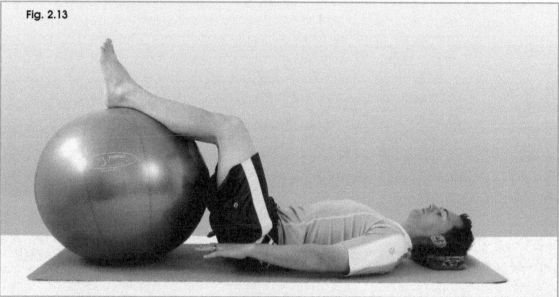

Fig. 2.13

movement 2: the hundred (breath only)

1. Leave the legs suspended over the ball and in good alignment. Keep the head down on the mat; focus only on the breath.

2. Inhale for five breaths through the nose and exhale for five breaths through the mouth. With each breath, gently pump your arms as if on a bed of springs. Reach with your fingers **(fig. 2.13)**.

3. Breathe for 80 to 100 counts.

4. For those students who may have a tendency to overarch the neck, a flat cushion can rest at the back of the skull and be used whenever you place your head on the mat.

Breath is regarded by many movement teachers as a crucial starting point, not only to better oxygenation but, as you will see in the next chapter, to stabilization. Here we will use the exhalation to activate the deep abdominals and other core muscles to ensure that the pelvis and low back are in a safe and secure position before and during movement. True functional strength is a harmonious blend of stability, strength, and mobility—some Pilates teachers refer to it as "moving stability." This fundamental concept will be thoroughly explored in the next chapter.

Check-In: The Right Ball for You

You have read through the chapter, understand the importance of the breath to focus the mind and relax the body, and are anxious to begin. But with so many balls on the market you may be confused about what ball, and what size, to choose. How hard or soft? And how do you blow up the ball and take care of it?

The appropriate size of ball to use is a subject of debate among teachers and depends on what exercise method you will be using. In Strength Training on the Ball we are not doing much bouncing on the ball, so I find the 55-centimeter ball to be a good size for most students, with the exception of those who are very tall (and strong). The larger the ball, the heavier and more unwieldy it is. A general rule is that when sitting on the ball the hips and knees should be bent at as close to a 90-degree angle as possible. This usually translates to 55-centimeter balls for people 5' to 5'8" and 65-centimeter balls for those who are 5'8" to 6'2".

Some exercises use different size balls for best results. The small ball shown in this chapter is a 9-inch Overball. Made in the Ledraplastic factory in Italy, the Overball has a pliable, skinlike surface; it can be used in place of the Pilates Circle or small Barrel to support or stretch the body. Overballs are weight-tested to 440 pounds (200 kilograms) and are inflated with a straw. A chi ball, a soft child's ball called a Gertie, or a large square or round piece of foam will work just as well.

Exercise balls are inexpensive and widely available in health and fitness shops. I personally prefer the Italian-made Fitballs (see page 259 for ordering information). I only use Fitballs in my teaching and personal workout because they have a surface that is not dangerously slippery but is pliable and firm without being heavy. Most important of all, they are burst resistant—essential when doing weight training on balls. If you accidentally roll over a small rock or tack they will not explode—they will deflate gradually. Fitballs have a faint and pleasant vanilla aroma, not a strong vinyl smell. They are latex-free and weight-tested to 1,000 pounds (455 kilograms) for normal use.

Beginners may find it easier to use a slightly underinflated ball, which will provide a larger base of support than a fully inflated ball does. If you are doing a lot of sitting or bouncing on the ball, then a firm ball, sized correctly, is desirable. If space allows it would be ideal to have balls of different sizes and degrees of softness: a soft ball is ideal for stretching whereas a firm ball is better for weight training and balance work.

Exercise balls are blown up according to diameter (height off the floor), not air pressure. A yardstick will help you inflate to the maximum diameter; the diameter is printed on the ball and on the box in which the ball is sold. Inflate only to the recommended diameter, not bigger. Most people find that a bicycle pump is not forceful enough. Use a raft or mattress pump or go to a gas station and use a cone-shaped trigger nozzle. I use a small inexpensive plastic pump that is totally portable and very effective for inflating the ball.

Practical Tips

- Comfortable yet fitted clothing is best for this work. Take care that clothing and hair are not too loose—both can get caught under the ball.
- A "less is more" approach applies to this method. If you have pain, you are pushing yourself too hard.
- An optimal workout schedule is three times a week, thirty minutes each session.
- It is not advisable to exercise after a meal.
- Start gradually. Be sure you have drinking water handy.
- Bare feet connect best with the floor. If you still find your feet slipping, use rubber-soled shoes.
- Work on a sticky yoga mat or a slip-resistant rug. Because the Pilates method involves rolling through the spine, place your yoga mat on a rug or a foam mat to provide cushioning for the spine.
- Be sure to have plenty of space around you.
- Check that the area is clear of staples, small stones, or other objects that may damage the ball.
- Read all the instructions thoroughly, paying close attention to the watchpoints.
- Check with your doctor or health practitioner to be sure these exercises are suitable for you. Pay attention to modifications and stop if there is any discomfort. If in doubt, avoid an exercise.

3

Stability Before Strength

Stability results from the stiffness at each joint in a particular degree of freedom.
—Stuart McGill, Ph.D.,
Low Back Disorders

Dawn's Story: Achieving "Moving Stability"

In her midforties Dawn, a nurse and an avid runner and hiker, was summoned to aid a choking woman. Her own mother had recently died and Dawn could not accept the fact that she could not save the 170-pound woman. She wrapped her arms around the woman's waist and attempted a last-resort effort: the Heimlich maneuver. The next day Dawn's upper back and midback were in spasm and she could not get out of bed.

An overachiever and a woman devoted to physical activity, Dawn dutifully did the circuit of physical therapists and chiropractors. After a period of time the injury appeared to be healed but she experienced recurring pain.

No place in the body is the phenomenon of "moving stability" more apparent than in the shoulder area, the place of the most mobile joints in the body. The shoulder blades must be free to move on the back of the rib cage but they must not move too far. According to Dawn's chiropractor, her serratus anterior, the broad muscle originating at the ribs and running to the shoulder blade, was weak. The serratus anterior and parts of the trapezius contract simultaneously to maintain the best placement of the shoulder blades. In addition, deep and superficial shoulder-joint muscles reinforce the capsule of the arm's ball and socket and keep the head of the arm bone in the proper position in the socket during arm movements.

The neck, upper back, and shoulders are closely related: when one is aberrant it affects the whole area.

In the lower half of Dawn's body something else was happening. All the years of backpacking and running had made Dawn what her chiropractor referred to as "bottom heavy" in her muscles. Unlike her upper body, which was relatively weak, her lower body was extremely strong—and tight. For years she had overworked the muscles of her hips, pelvis, and low back: the results—too much stiffness, too little movement, and a propensity toward spasms. It was as if Dawn couldn't get her lower body to turn off—a dominant movement habit that had been going on for years. Her nervous system fired in the same habitual way as it always had, making the strong muscles stronger and the weak muscles weaker. Dawn reminded me of other athletes with whom I have worked whose tightness and stiffness do not allow for sufficient movement in the joints. Some bodybuilders are so developed in the shoulders and chest that the arms appear to be fused in their joints. Sometimes laborers who use their lower body, hips, and pelvis for lifting and manual labor can become so tight in the hips and low back that they lose much of the natural spring necessary in the joints. It is not only tight muscles that affect mobility—rigidity in the fascia, tendons, and joint capsules can lead to the same result.

Dawn confessed that in the beginning she couldn't even balance on the ball and kept rolling off. She knew her balance abilities were weak, but working out with a ball brought that awareness home for her in a way a mat or a machine would not have. On the ball she had to keep good form: she couldn't "cheat" (she would roll off of the ball) and, most important of all, she could not rush through the exercises.

During the first five weeks of working on the ball, Dawn's balance and flexibility improved radically and she began to stretch out the large and small muscles and the connective tissue of the pelvis, hip, and legs to achieve more mobility. Most important of all, she no longer had pain in her upper back. By working with smaller rather than larger weights she learned to "turn on" her shoulder stabilizers and provide support for arm movements.

"Big Engines" Versus "Control Engines"

In contrast to traditional body-conditioning methods, which isolate the outer and more visible superficial muscles of the arms, chest, back, and legs, Pilates-based strength training focuses on the deep inner layer—the stabilizers. This is what makes Strength Training on the Ball different from other approaches. Generally, stabilizers (sometimes called postural muscles) are designed to contract for sustained periods of time to provide support for mobility. Usually they are deep muscles (though in the shoulder area they are not as deep or as small as in the spine and pelvis) and are associated with acts of endurance. They contract more slowly than mobilizers but keep you erect and moving for a long period of time. Think of a spaceship: it is the big engines that function during blast off, yet it is the control engines that operate with precision to dock the ship in space. When working properly these small, deep muscles known as the stabilizers fix the spinal joints safely in place and support the bone in the socket or joint.

Mobilizers, on the other hand, are designed for one-off, powerful movements of brief duration such as bending the spine forward, backward, or sideways. These superficial muscles work in a large range of motion, but they burn out quickly. The tricep is a "blast-off" muscle and when it is stressed with resistance the tricep will grow bigger and more shapely. However, at the same time as the tricep is being pumped up, other muscles—the stabilizers—are at work to keep the shoulder blades in place, to maintain the correct position of the arm in the socket, and to ensure that the spine is erect and in good posture. As the triceps work to straighten the arm, the rotator cuff muscles control the shoulder joint and the serratus anterior and parts of the trapezius stabilize the shoulder blades.

If a deep stabilizer is not toned and functioning properly, a mobilizer may take over the stabilizer's job. For example, whenever the deep stabilizing rhomboid muscles around Dawn's shoulder blades and the serratus anterior, under her armpit, did not work correctly, the upper trapezius and neck muscles went into spasm as did some spinal mobilizers.

According to Stuart McGill, Ph.D., a leading expert on spine function and injury prevention, all of the trunk muscles contribute to stabilization and it may be a mistake to target one single type of muscle as being more important than another. Different muscles in the stability formula can modulate between tasks as demands and constraints are placed on them. When you raise a heavy bag of potatoes from the ground it is the mobilizers that allow you to straighten up. Yet it is the stabilizers that enable you to stand without falling over as they work in relays to keep you erect. The stabilizers work automatically in a person with a healthy back. Pain and problems occur when the stabilizers are not functioning properly toward fulfilling their correct tasks. Perhaps initially you hold the bag of potatoes in your arms and feel no pain. However, if you stand or walk with a bag of potatoes in your arms you will need to take frequent rests—and you may even experience pain—because the mobilizers, not designed to hold the body up for periods of time, can work as stabilizers but they rapidly burn out when they are not fulfilling their proper role. Mobilizers burn out quicker because they have mainly fast-twitch fibers and work at a fuller capacity than the stabilizers, which are designed for endurance and control rather than strength.

To achieve the goal of "moving stability," all systems in the body—including bone, muscle, and breath—must work together to build a strong and functional organism. Cooperation should develop as body awareness increases. And it is the nervous system that has a major role to play in this body awareness.

Nervous-System Error

When the nervous system works efficiently it activates just the right muscles at the right time to protect the spine or other joints for movement. What happens if the nervous system fails to correctly activate the proper muscles when necessary?

Sensory nerves carry to the brain information about what is happening in the body and in the area around it. As a person bends to pick up the bag of potatoes, the central nervous system sends an order signaling the muscle fibers to contract in a certain way to "meet" the situation. Think of the nervous system as a computer: if the computer is not programmed properly the appropriate muscles may fail to activate adequately. This nervous-system error could cause a joint in the spine to be injured if the deep stabilizers don't fire—if they fail to create the protective "stiffness" needed before a person reaches for the bag or moves the bag from one position to the next. Dr. Stuart McGill and his colleagues studied various bending-and-lifting scenarios, some of their subjects lifting heavy loads and others lifting very light loads. They concluded that back injury can occur even in the most innocent task, such as picking a pencil off the floor. Suddenly, as the person reaches for the pencil, there is an error in the muscle control and one tiny portion of the spine rotates to a point that irritation or injury occurs. Previous injuries, muscle imbalances, and faulty breathing patterns can all contribute to nervous-system error and faulty motor control.

By now you understand that in a Pilates approach to strength training we are greatly concerned that the stabilizers are toned and programmed properly to provide support for mobility. But if there is a neurological inability to fire the correct muscle, ordinary strengthening exercises will not help. To correct nervous-system error you need to begin from scratch, possibly with the help of an expert in spinal stabilization, to reprogram the body so you have better control of the deepest layer of your body.

Precise movement is dependent upon constant accurate messaging to and from the brain—this is why nervous-system training is an important aspect of exercise. There is evidence that working on a moving surface such as a ball wakes up inactive motor units and inspires them to fire more successfully. (Inactive motor units are part of the muscular fiber of the muscle which, because they are not needed, are not activated by the nervous system. The body is lazy and only works as much as it has to, nothing more.) Working on a mobile surface continuously throws the body off balance and forces your brain to confront the unfamiliar and ever-changing. Sensory nerves become better trained and can more rapidly send messages to your brain. The brain in turn processes information quicker and sends messages to the muscles faster, improving reaction time. When this happens the body can organize itself better for function and power. This is helpful not only in sports but in daily life—think about the times that you've not hurt yourself by catching a railing as you felt your feet going out from under you.

Thomas Hanna's groundbreaking 1988 book *Somatics* is about reestablishing the mind's control of the body. His premise is that malfunctions of the sensorimotor system cause deterioration, stiffness, and pain. He believes that sensorimotor deficiencies should be solved not only by the doctor or practitioner but by the patient teaching him- or herself to gain control of the body by being shown how a certain muscular pattern feels. "Sensory awareness of the muscles goes hand in hand with voluntary motor control of the muscles," writes Hanna. "If you cannot sense it, you cannot move it, and the more you can move it, the more you will sense it."

Balls and Rehabilitation

how exactly does a therapist use a ball to rehabilitate an adult?

Movement begins in the frontal cortex of the brain. An impaired central nervous system affects the muscles' abilities to contract properly, but the challenge and unfamiliarity of the ball forces the brain to stay active. Thus there is growing evidence that the nervous system greatly benefits from ballwork.

In Beate Carrière's definitive textbook for using balls for rehabilitation, *The Swiss Ball: Theory, Basic Exercises, and Clinical Application*, she describes how a ball can be used to test and improve range of movement, strength, balance, alignment, and proprioception in back patients. The flexibility of the ball means a therapist can also use the ball to rehabilitate an injured or replaced knee, hip, or shoulder, even in a hospital bed. The ball elevates the affected limb; the patient is challenged to keep the leg or arm aligned while increasing the range of movement, working the good side first and then the weak side. Most important, the patient is in control of the movement.

The Pre-Pilates Stabilizing Exercises

The pre-Pilates exercises are not strength exercises as we generally know them. We start at a low level of intensity. We use the work of attention to reeducate the body and, if necessary, the nervous system so that the stabilizers of the low back and abdomen, primarily the transversus abdominis, pelvic floor, and lumbar multifidus, are working together to withstand movements of limbs and the spine. We do this by putting the body through precise movement patterns and repeating them enough times so they become ingrained in the body's muscle memory. If you have chronic back problems, read the section on low-back pain in chapter 8 and learn about the current research on low-back instability and nervous-system error that is coming out of Queensland, Australia. Then, I highly recommend you locate a good physical therapist or personal trainer, one who is familiar with spinal stabilization, to make sure you are performing the exercises correctly.

To reprogram the body so that there is a balance between stability and mobility, a "less is more" approach is best. A lot of effort is *not* necessary. Overtensing can distort the body, pulling it out of alignment and encouraging the wrong muscles to fire. Instead of working for large movements or powerful contractions, in Strength Training on the Ball we work with low-level, gentle, precise movements. Modest levels of activation with an equal co-contraction of the opposite muscles will create more than adequate stability in most people.

In many ways the exercises in this chapter are the most important ones in the book. They prepare you for everything else that follows while at the same time reviewing key goals and principles. Unfortunately, I can see people skipping ahead, thinking "these are too easy for me." On the contrary, these exercises are not at all simple and it may be necessary to call in an expert to help you. Remember: if your computer is not programmed correctly you will encounter problems, sometimes serious ones, later on. So it is with the body and the balance between the stabilizers and the mobilizers.

Be patient. Most of us are not used to training the invisible, inner-layer muscles. "Why am I not sweating?" some people will demand. "How will Heel Slides give me more defined buttocks?" They won't. Training of the more flashy outer layer of muscles can be added to a fitness program once the deep stabilizers have been located and rehabilitated to provide support for the low back and pelvis. As some types of therapeutic exercises are more compatible than others, take this book with you to your physical therapist and ask which exercises may be suitable for you.

repetition creates habit

Stuart McGill reminds us: "Practice does not make perfect, it makes permanent." This can lead to two radically different approaches when trying to achieve "moving stability." If you practice exercises in good motion patterns, with a clear memory pathway, you will activate the correct muscles to create stability in the desired area.

A clear memory pathway means that accurate messages are getting to and from the brain. The goal is to create and reinforce a movement pattern that allows your body to work efficiently. At first a new (correct) pattern may feel wrong, yet eventually the movement pattern will become automatic.

What happens, however, when you push the body too far too fast and repeat movement habits that don't allow your body to move correctly? In this case, faulty practice grooves faulty motor patterns, and it takes much longer to undo these patterns than it took to establish them in the first place.

Repetition creates habit. This is why it is important to slow down and focus your attention when you are learning new exercises.

Navel-to-Spine

Kneeling on all fours is an effective position to practice keeping the spine stabilized and the abdominals connected while adding small movement of the limbs. To keep the abdominals connected means to tighten them by using the exhalation to gently draw the area between the pubic bone and navel toward the spine. Later you will also learn to engage the pelvic floor, the sling of muscles between your pubic bone and tailbone, but for now just focus on finding the connection in the deep abdominals without allowing any movement in the pelvis or spine. This contraction should be very small and precise, with the buttocks remaining relaxed. Think of executing this contraction in the same way as you would work a dimmer switch—slowly and gently draw tension into the abdominals. Do not suck in the belly, which will activate the more superficial layer of musculature. Try the movement first without the ball and then place your belly on a large soggy ball that does not compress your chest or rib cage. In movement 3, hold the contraction in the abdominals for five seconds, breathing naturally. This contraction will develop strength and endurance in the stabilizers.

Purpose To learn how to create a strong center by gently drawing the navel in toward the spine.

Watchpoints • The action of drawing the navel up and toward the spine is small and subtle. • Think of gently drawing inward the area between the pubic bone and navel. • The buttocks muscles are not involved. • Avoid arching or rounding the back or moving the pelvis in any way. • Inhale through the nose and exhale through the mouth, sending the breath into the back of the rib cage. • Avoid holding your breath.

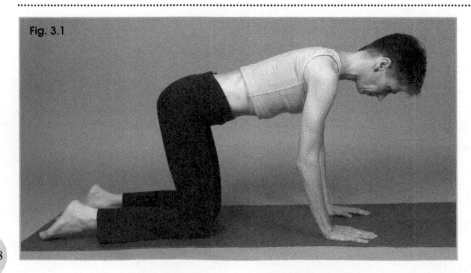

Fig. 3.1

starting position

Begin on all fours, taking care to make sure your hands are aligned below the shoulders and your knees are aligned below the hip joints **(fig. 3.1)**. Your weight is equally distributed on all four limbs; knees are apart. Lengthen through the back of the neck so the crown of your head moves away from your tailbone. The gaze is on the mat. The spine is in neutral, not arched or too flat. Elbows are soft, not locked.

movement 1: stabilizing on all fours

1. Let your belly gently release with gravity without moving the spine or pelvis. Take a few easy, relaxing breaths **(fig. 3.2)**.

2. On the exhalation gently draw the navel up toward the spine. There should be no movement in either the spine or the pelvis **(fig. 3.3)**.

3. Inhale to release the navel.

4. Exhale to lift the navel gently upward. Think of drawing the area between the pubic bone and the navel toward the spine.

5. Inhale to release.

6. Repeat six times. Do not hold your breath.

movement 2: with ball

1. Lie over a slightly underinflated large ball. Do not let the round shape of the ball distract you from maintaining a neutral back. This means do not collapse over the ball but instead lengthen through the spine. Hands are directly beneath the shoulders, knees beneath the hips. Depending on the size of the ball you may have your weight on your toes rather than your knees.

2. Inhale to lengthen through the spine.

3. Exhale to gently draw your navel up toward your spine **(fig. 3.4)**.

4. Inhale to release your navel onto the ball. Repeat this movement five times.

movement 3: add hold

1. Begin in the same position as movement 2. Inhale to lengthen through the spine.

2. Exhale to gently draw your navel upward. Keep a slight tension in the abdominals as you breathe in and out for 3 to 5 counts.

3. Repeat this movement five times.

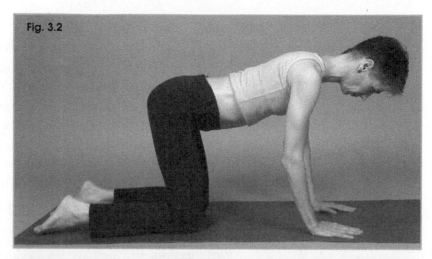

Fig. 3.2

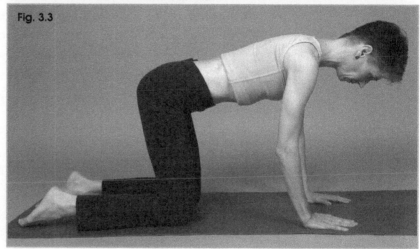

Fig. 3.3

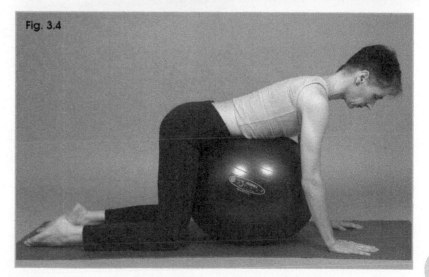

Fig. 3.4

Tailbone Curls

Finding and maintaining neutral pelvis is a key goal in the Pilates Method. Neutral pelvis stabilizes the low back and places the vertebral discs in a safe, uncompressed position. In Tailbone Curls we use the abdominal muscles to move the pelvis in and out of neutral. This movement may help some students find their neutral-pelvis position. Depending on the shape of your body and buttocks, when your pelvis is in the neutral position you may be able to ease your fingers into the space between the low back and the floor. It is desirable that the space here be smaller rather than gaping.

Purpose To locate neutral pelvis and draw awareness to the pelvis and low back.

Watchpoints • If you have low-back pain, avoid overarching or overflattening the back—keep the tilt small. • Try not to create tension in any other part of the body. • Neither the buttocks nor the thigh muscles should be working in this exercise. • Relax them. • Use the abdominals to tilt the pelvis. • Remember to inhale into the back rib cage.

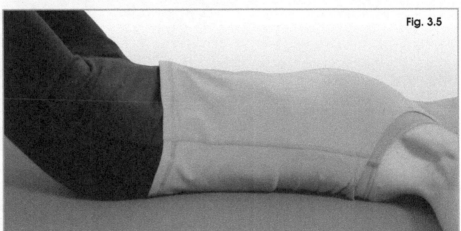

Fig. 3.5

starting position

Lie on your back with your knees bent. Feet should be hip-distance apart and parallel, in line with your knees. The knees are in line with your hips.

movement: tilting the pelvis in and out of neutral

1. Inhale. Exhale to gently pull in the muscles of the low abdomen, slightly tilting the pelvis and flattening the low back against the mat. The pubic bone will lift **(fig. 3.5)**.

2. Inhale to drop your pubic bone downward so that there is a slope run-

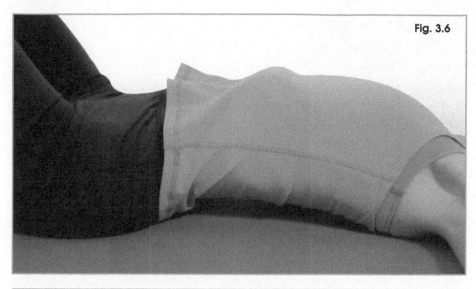

Fig. 3.6

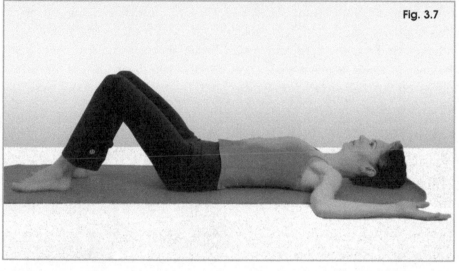

Fig. 3.7

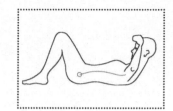

neutral pelvis

Neutral pelvis is the balance between low back and pelvis, a position that stabilizes the low back and places the discs in a safe, uncompressed position. We take the body as it is standing up, with its natural curves in the back, and simply lie it down on the mat.

Some teachers teach neutral pelvis by having their students lie down and locate the hipbones and pubic bone on the front of the pelvis to see if they are in the same plane. This works if you have a conventional body. Another approach is to imagine a heaviness at the base of the sacrum, the triangular bone at the base of the spine. There will be a slight curve; you may be able to ease your fingers into the space between your low back and the floor—but you may not, too, depending on shape of body and buttocks. It is always desirable that this space be smaller rather than gaping.

ning from the hipbones on the front of your pelvis to your pubic bone. You will feel an exaggerated arch in your back **(fig. 3.6)**.

3. Repeat several times, gently tilting the pelvis in both directions.

4. Finish by allowing the pelvis to rest in neutral. The tailbone should feel heavy as it lengthens on the mat. Your pelvis is neither tipped up nor dropped downward **(fig. 3.7)**.

Pelvic Floor and Knee-Lift Stabilizing Exercise

Place your calves on a ball and try to relax the back of the legs and low back. The goal in movement 1 of this series is to activate the muscles of the pelvic floor. Located on the bottom of the pelvis, the pelvic floor connects through the nervous system to the deep abdominal muscles. Without allowing the tailbone to lift off the mat or the gluteals to tighten, you should feel the pelvic-floor muscles, especially the front portion, gently squeeze together as the bottom of the pelvis draws up. Imagine you have an extremely full bladder and are tightening these muscles to stop the flow of urine as you search for a bathroom. Women may recognize this movement as a Kegel exercise. In movement 2, for a few seconds hold the pelvic-floor contraction without holding your breath. Then in movement 3 place your three longest fingers one inch inside your hipbones and press in gently yet deeply. With the correct "dimmer switch" contraction you will feel a continual subtle tension in your fingertips as the transversus abdominis flattens. If you feel a muscle bulge up into your fingers rather than flatten, it is probably a more superficial abdominal—the oblique—and not the deep transversus. In movement 4 you will try to keep the deep abdominal–pelvic-floor connection as you slowly lift one knee two inches off the ball. Initiate from the hip, however, not from the knee, to ensure that this is not just a bend and stretch of the knee.

Purpose To locate the deep abdominal connection and pelvic floor and to feel how the pelvic-floor contraction triggers the deep abdominals.

Watchpoints • Do not let the pelvis move or tilt. • The buttocks should be relaxed. • In movement 4, keep the knee lift small. • Keep the tailbone heavy on the mat.

....

starting position

Lie on your back. Place the legs up on the ball and relax the head and shoulders on the mat.

movement 1: locating the pelvic floor

1. Take a few easy breaths to relax.
2. On the exhalation slowly contract the pelvic floor, gently drawing it upward. Imagine you are attempting to stop the

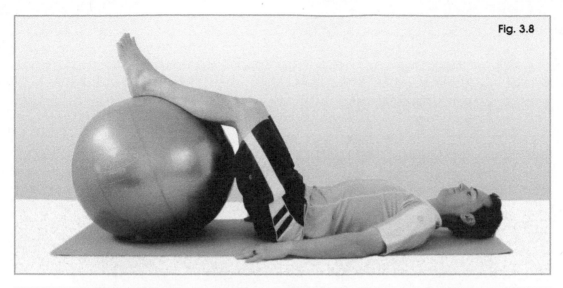

Fig. 3.8

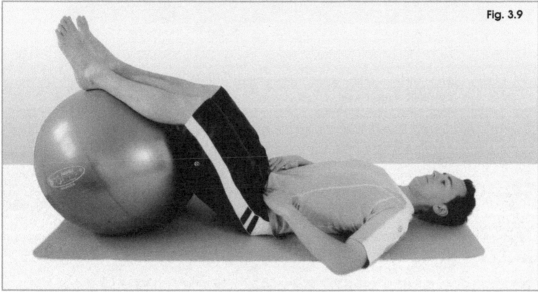

Fig. 3.9

flow of urine. Keep your pelvis in neutral, buttocks relaxed **(fig. 3.8)**.

3. Inhale to release the pelvic floor.

4. Without holding your breath, exhale to tighten the pelvic floor.

5. Repeat four times.

movement 2: add hold

1. Take a few easy breaths to relax.

2. On the exhalation slowly contract the pelvic floor, gently drawing it upward. Imagine you are attempting to stop the

flow of urine. Keep your pelvis in neutral, buttocks relaxed.

3. Hold for 3 to 5 seconds. Breathe naturally.

4. Gradually relax the pelvic floor.

5. Repeat four times.

movement 3: feel the transversus abdominis

1. Place your three longest fingers one inch in from your hipbones and press in gently yet deeply **(fig. 3.9)**. Take a few easy breaths to relax.

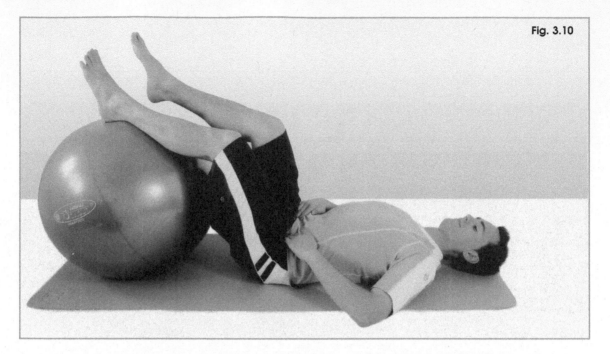

Fig. 3.10

2. On the exhalation slowly contract the pelvic floor, gently drawing it upward. Imagine you are attempting to stop the flow of urine. Keep your pelvis in neutral, buttocks relaxed. Do not hold your breath.

3. Can you feel the subtle pressure on your fingertips as the pelvic floor contraction activates the transversus abdominis? You should feel the muscle flatten rather than bulge up into your fingertips.

4. Hold for 3 to 5 seconds, breathing naturally. Gradually relax the pelvic-floor contraction. Repeat four times.

movement 4: single-knee lift

1. Place your fingertips one inch in from your hipbones and press in gently but deeply. Inhale to prepare.

2. Exhale to draw in your lower abdomen, pull up the pelvic floor, and find the contraction of the deep transversus abdominis muscle.

3. Inhale to keep the contraction. You should continue to feel tension in your fingertips.

4. Exhale to lift the right knee two inches off the ball **(fig. 3.10)**.

5. Inhale to stay.

6. Exhale to slowly place the right leg back on the ball, keeping the abdominal connection.

7. Alternate legs. Repeat four times each leg.

Heel Slides and Single-Leg Circles

These exercises are not as easy as they look. They help us make a distinction between pelvis and leg, to remind us of the joint that joins the two. Use the deep abdominals and the pelvic floor to try to keep the pelvis calm and anchored and in neutral position while the thigh bone moves smoothly in its ball and socket. In Single-Leg Circles you could use a resistance band at the back of the thigh to help guide the leg. Hold the band in your hands and angle the arms down and slightly open on the mat to release the shoulders. Keep the wrists straight and not bent at the crease. Movements 4 and 5 are more challenging as the supporting leg is placed on the mobile ball and will show any wobbling in the pelvis. Keep the circling knee bent to begin with; eventually the leg can straighten.

Purpose To keep the pelvis stable and in neutral while the limbs move freely.

Watchpoints • The foot stays on the mat in Heel Slides. • Keep the knee bent in Single-Leg Circles and ensure that the toes are softly pointed, not locked into a tense ballet pointe. • Use the navel-to-spine connection to keep the pelvis steady, anchored, and in neutral.

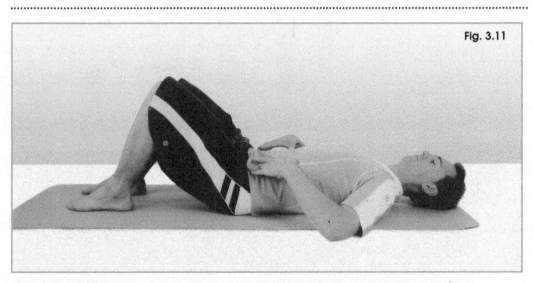

Fig. 3.11

starting position
Lie on your back with your knees bent. The feet should be hip-distance apart and parallel, in line with your knees; knees are in line with your hips. Place your thumb on the bottom of your rib cage and your three longest fingers on your hipbones to make sure there is no pelvic movement forward or backward or from side to side as you perform this exercise **(fig. 3.11)**.

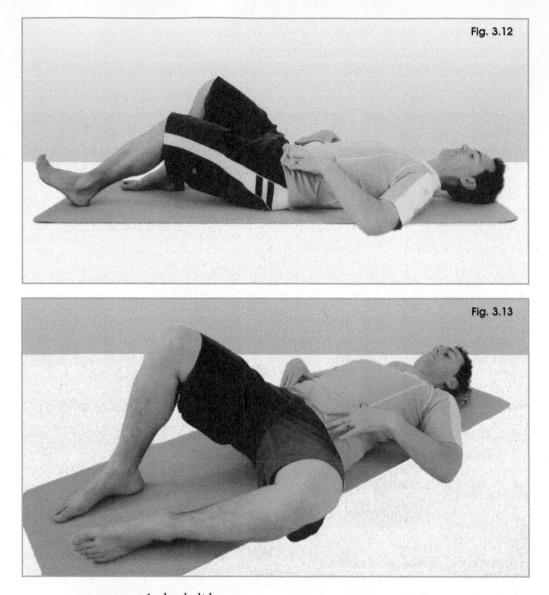

Fig. 3.12

Fig. 3.13

movement 1: heel slides

1. Inhale to prepare.

2. On the exhalation slowly contract the pelvic floor, gently drawing it upward as you slowly slide away the left leg along the mat. Keep the pelvis still as you slide the leg halfway down the length of the mat **(fig. 3.12)**.

3. Inhale to pause, keeping the abdominal connection.

4. Exhale to slide the left leg back to the starting position.

5. Repeat three to five times and repeat on the other side.

movement 2: open knee

1. Inhale to prepare.

2. On the exhalation slowly contract the pelvic floor, gently drawing it upward as you open the left knee away from the midline **(fig. 3.13)**. Keep the pelvis still and only allow the knee to fall to the side as far as you can while still keeping the pelvis steady. This will not be very far.

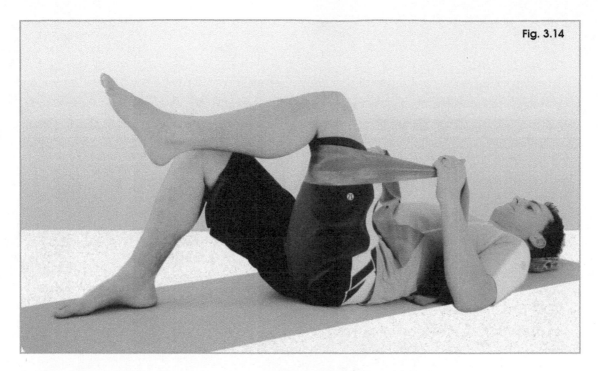

Fig. 3.14

3. Inhale at the bottom of the movement, maintaining the abdominal connection.

4. Exhale to return the leg to the starting position.

5. Repeat three to five times and then perform the movement on the other side.

movement 3: small single-leg circles

1. If desired, use a resistance band across the back of the thigh. Hold the band in your hands, elbows down on the mat. Inhale and exhale to peel the leg up. The knee will be bent and directly above your hip **(fig. 3.14)**.

2. Imagine you are drawing a circle in the direction of the ceiling with your kneecap. Inhaling for half the circle and exhaling for the other half, make sure you brush through all quarter positions of a clock's face: three o'clock,

six o'clock, nine o'clock, twelve o'clock. Keep the pelvis stable as you circle.

3. Do five circles clockwise, inhaling for half the circle, exhaling for the other half of the circle.

4. Do five circles counterclockwise, inhaling for half the circle, exhaling for the other half of the circle.

5. Now repeat on the opposite leg.

movement 4: single-leg circles on ball

1. Place your supporting leg on the ball as if it were the floor. If desired, place your thumbs on the bottom of your rib cage and your three longest fingers on your hipbones to make sure there is no movement forward or backward or from side to side in the pelvis as you practice this exercise. Press the ball out slightly so that it is not too close to your body. Keep the pelvis in neutral as you

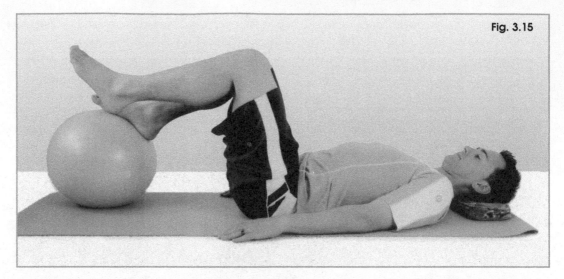

Fig. 3.15

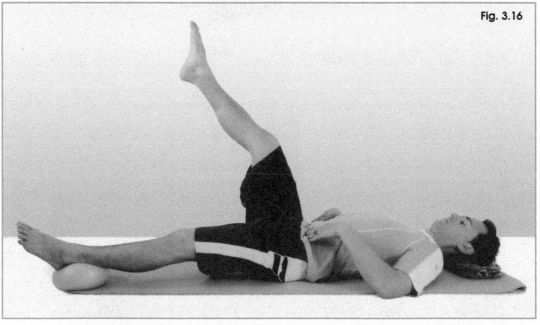

Fig. 3.16

lift one knee to the twelve o'clock position **(fig. 3.15)**.

2. As in movement 3, do five circles in each direction and repeat on the opposite leg.

movement 5: single-leg circles on small ball

1. Straighten the supporting leg and place it on the small ball. If desired, place your thumbs on the bottom of your rib cage and your three longest fingers on your hipbones to make sure there is no movement forward or backward or from side to side in the pelvis **(fig. 3.16)**. Or just slide the fingers down the mat.

2. As above, do five circles in each direction and repeat on the opposite leg.

3. Use the navel-to-spine contraction to keep the pelvis steady.

Scapula Isolation and Rib Cage Stability

The shoulder blades at the back of the rib cage need to be stabilized before you move the arms or lift the upper body off the mat. Think of the shoulder blades as gently sliding down the back because if they are up by your ears you will create tension in the neck and upper shoulders. Movement 1 shows you how to isolate the shoulder blades by lifting them up and gently setting them back into place. When they are properly in place they are in the right position to allow the arm to move freely and safely. The ball gives you a gentle weight to work with, but don't let the ball drift back toward your head. Keep it above your breastbone and keep widening across the front of the collarbones. In movement 2 we use the abdominals to stabilize the rib cage when taking the arms overhead. Pay attention that the back is not arching off the mat and the ribs are not popping open.

Purpose To consciously feel the movement in the shoulder blades and to learn to release the blades gently into the mat. Movement 2 teaches stability in the rib cage while elevating the arms.

Watchpoints • Keep widening across the front of the collarbones. In movement 2, don't take the ball too far overhead—the arms will be extended but soft at the elbows. • Use the abdominals to keep the rib cage from "popping" and the back from arching off the mat.

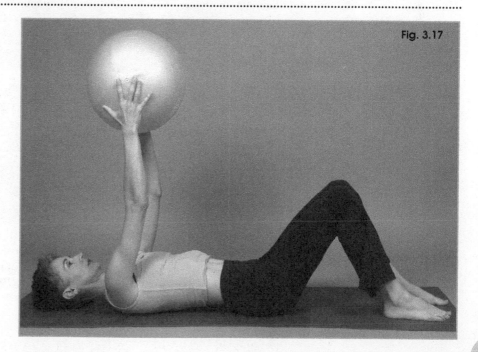

Fig. 3.17

starting position

Lie on your back with your legs straight or bent. Hold the ball on the sides above your chest. Make sure your elbows are soft, not hyperextended.

movement 1: scapula isolation

1. Inhale to reach your fingertips toward the ceiling, lifting the shoulder blades slightly off the mat **(fig. 3.17)**.
2. Exhale to lower the shoulder

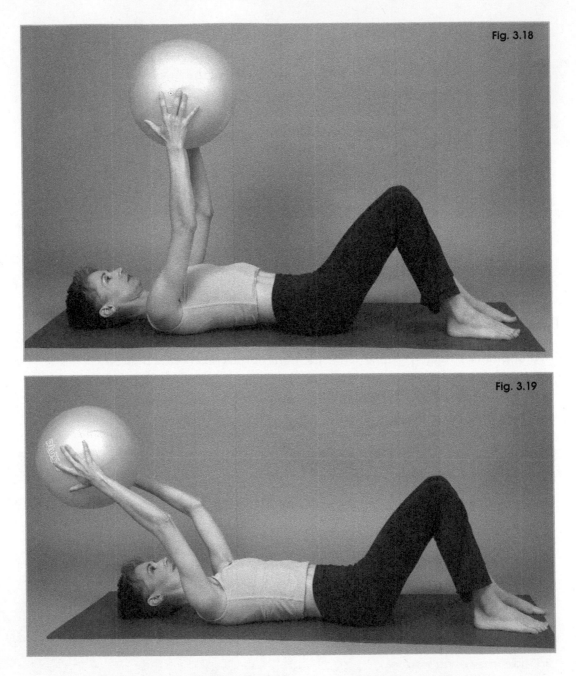

Fig. 3.18

Fig. 3.19

blades to neutral position **(fig. 3.18)**.
3. Repeat three to five times.

movement 2: rib cage stability

1. From the same starting position, inhale to prepare.
2. Exhale to sink the navel toward the spine and to take the ball slightly overhead, keeping the rib cage from popping out or the back from arching **(fig. 3.19)**.
3. Inhale to lift the ball and place it over the breastbone.
4. Repeat three to five times.

Half Roll-Downs with Resistance Band

In this exercise, adapted from the Pilates Cadillac apparatus, you have an opportunity to practice gently drawing the navel in toward the spine, engaging the pelvic floor, and releasing the pelvis away from the legs. Review the safety sidebar for using resistance bands, and make sure the resistance band is carefully and widely wrapped across the back of your feet. Work at using the abdominals and releasing through the top of the thighs to ensure that the deep thigh muscles are not overworking. Keep the knees bent and feet flexed as you sit up tall on your sitz bones. To find the sitz bones, or ischial tuberosities, place your hand under one buttock and move the fleshy part to the side. Palpate the rocker on the bottom of your pelvis; begin this exercise by sitting up tall and evenly on these rockers.

Purpose To practice drawing the navel gently into the spine and rolling back while maintaining the abdominal connection.

Watchpoints • Release the shoulders. • Keep the feet flexed and the knees bent.

....

starting position

Sit up on your sitz bones with your knees bent and your feet hip-distance apart. Carefully wrap the resistance band across the back of your flexed feet, keeping the band wide. Hold the band.

movement: half roll-down

1. Inhale to sit tall, reaching through the tips of your ears toward the ceiling **(fig. 3.20)**.

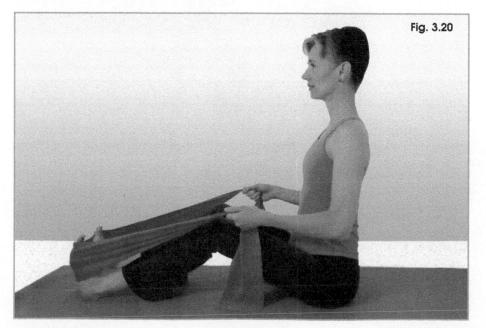

Fig. 3.20

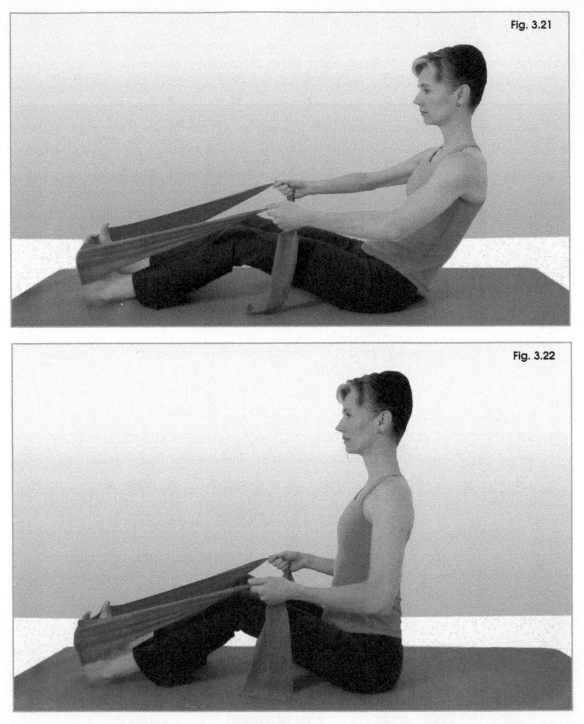

Fig. 3.21

Fig. 3.22

2. Exhale to draw your navel to your spine and roll back off your sitz bones **(fig. 3.21)**.

3. Inhale to curl forward and then roll up tall onto the sitz bones **(fig. 3.22)**. Repeat five times.

Safety Precautions for Use of Resistance Bands

resistance bands have a close association with Pilates exercises because of how the resistance of the band stimulates spring tension of the Pilates equipment. They are very effective for upper- and lower-body work, but it is important to consider how the elastic material works and how to set the body up best to benefit from the unique properties of elasticity.

Elastic resistance bands are produced by various manufacturers in an assortment of thicknesses that provide different levels of resistance. They are usually about 10 centimeters wide and color coded to let you know their degree of resistance. Try to maintain the full width of the band whenever possible to prevent the band from digging into hands or slipping off your feet. If the band pulls on your leg hair, wear long socks. A length of 5 feet is good for Pilates-based resistance work. Inspect your band frequently and replace it if you notice nicks. Beware of long fingernails when you hold the band and jagged toenails during exercises where you wrap the band across the soles of the feet. Store the band out of direct sunlight and away from heat sources. Replace it frequently.

The resistance band should be taut but not too stretched out when you begin. It is essential that you have a firm grip on the end of the band so that it does not snap back toward your eyes. Take care when looping the band across the feet that it does not fly back into your face. Resistance bands can cause injury if not used properly so I would not encourage their use with children. For patients in the hospital or rehabilation, who are doing exercises under the supervision of a physical therapist, make sure the band is securely tied to the frame of the hospital bed.

Optimal strength, fitness, and function depend on a balance between two forces: anchoring and mobility. The body is constantly changing and interacting with the demands of gravity; the next chapter will show you how to assess your posture and test your balance.

As you read through the check-in below, think about the words of international ballet star Margot Fonteyn: "Minor things can become moments of great revelation when encountered for the first time."

Check-In: The Work of Attention

"Attention is an act of will, of work against the inertia of our own minds," M. Scott Peck writes in his popular book *The Road Less Traveled*. The work of attention, attests Peck, nurtures our own or another's spiritual growth.

Once Dawn began to concentrate on correcting the imbalances in her body, she realized that in the past her workouts, like so many aspects of her life, were frenzied and fast paced: she focused on the distractions around her, not on the here and now of each movement. Now she was working slowly and with precision. In addition to nurturing spiritual growth, the work of attention is also essential for regulating and modifying structures of the physical body. Dawn confessed to me that one of the greatest differences in working with the ball was that she learned to slow down during exercise and use the work of attention to break the faulty but dominant movement patterns that controlled her body.

I experienced the rewards of focused attention long before I ever taught movement. This was during a particularly restless time in my life. I had too much energy—I could not sit still, my mind was spilling over with ideas for new projects, and yet I had volunteered to sit twice a week and listen to a foreign student struggle in English! The first time I took a deep breath, repressed the urge to interrupt, and simply listened, I was astonished by the results. I grew entirely calm and at peace, stimulated by the student's words. I listened to her as if in a trance and she responded to my stillness and attention by forming full, confident sentences. Since that time I have learned to apply the work of attention to my Pilates teaching.

The work of attention places you entirely in the moment, and marvelous things can happen there, both as a student and as a teacher. Suddenly every movement that is made, whether it is dropping the chin slightly or learning to draw up the pelvic floor, is part of the whole. Using the mind to sense what is going on in the body is a demanding task.

To benefit from the pre-Pilates exercises keep in mind the following:

1. *Remember the goal of this work: to use the mind to reeducate the body.* First we locate specific muscles with a small isolated contraction. Think of this contraction working like a "dimmer switch," the contraction will build slowly and subtly. Once this slow, deep contraction is found, then we add small movements.
2. *Concentration is essential.* Turn off music and other distractions to keep the mind from wandering away from the work. Try to work in an area where you will not be interrupted. Wear loose, comfortable clothing and stay relaxed.
3. *Make sure that you are not concentrating so hard that you forget to breathe.* Use the exhalation to activate the deep muscles and to release areas that

are overworking. Some physical therapists advocate passive breathing as the best way to rehabilitate the pelvic floor, transversus abdominis, and multifidus. This is a different approach from Pilates lateral breathing. Passive breathing is three-dimensional breathing with a relaxed belly, and some believe that this approach works best when learning to find the subtle "dimmer switch" contraction. Whatever breathing style you use, do not hold your breath.

4. *Take breaks and don't overdo it.* It's much harder to feel a subtle contraction than to feel a large one. In a squat series, the thighs will feel a burn and fatigue in a very obvious way. This is not the case in working with pelvic floor, deep abdominals, and other stabilizers.

5. *If at all possible, work with a qualified practitioner.* The pre-Pilates exercises are more mentally challenging than physically challenging. A physical therapist or a highly qualified personal trainer with experience in spinal stabilization will vary the position of the body and the pelvis to find out what is best for you to feel the subtle firing of the pelvic floor and deep abdominals. He or she will also be able to palpate your low back to test if the lumbar multifidus, the deep bands of muscles passing from one vertebra to another, are firing correctly. A dysfunctional multifidus is a common factor in low-back pain. Please see the section on low-back pain in chapter 8. A trained professional can help you feel the pelvic floor, transversus, and multifidus working together so you can build in the ability to create the "dimmer switch" contraction on your own.

4
Strength Training, Posture, and Balance

Often the body speaks clearly that which the tongue refuses to utter.
—Mabel E. Todd, *The Thinking Body*

Arthur's Story

Art couldn't remember when the limping began. It was not pronounced enough to think about using a cane—not yet: he was only sixty-eight—but he felt his body lurching slightly to the right now as he walked. His one leg felt as if it had trouble swinging through. It was as if his leg threw his body off balance, or maybe his body threw his leg off-kilter. He felt shortened down one side—it was either bad posture or natural aging, or both. In any case his step was heavy and had lost its spring.

In normal walking the foot hits the ground heel first and then the body's weight rolls through the foot. The muscles of the supporting arches of the feet contract as the foot comes into full contact with the ground. The knee ensures that the body's weight is lowered with control. The arms swing and the upper and lower body rotate freely. If the body's posture is stooped and the shoulders rounded or if the pelvis is not allowing the legs to swing evenly, one's sense of balance and confidence is compromised. The gait becomes slow, uneven, and heavy-footed.

Art had recently retired and according to him that was when all his troubles began. When he worked he often found himself irritable and stressed, yet now he sorely missed the action of the office. He couldn't really afford to retire but it was compulsory, so he was left helplessly fretting over investments and an unpredictable stock market. As a younger man he used to bury frustrations

56

into weekend hockey games and skiing, but he believed he was definitely too old for all that. Two years ago he took a fall while ice skating. He hurt his knee at that time and decided to stop skating all together. He went to a local gym but was unable to find a program that challenged him. When he told his wife he had enrolled in a class working out with large balls, she wondered whatever had put that idea into his head. She was afraid he would roll off the ball and hurt himself.

Studies of movement and aging indicate that falling is a result of decreased strength and mobility. The more inactive one is, the more the skills needed to keep the body safely upright are diminished. In Art's case, the curtailment of skating and other activities he loved meant less practice with balance and a concomitant loss of confidence in navigating himself through his daily activities.

The truth is, as aging adults we need more practice in falling—not less—but falling within safe boundaries.

Pilates on the ball did not solve all of Art's problems, but his balance improved considerably and his body keenly needed the deep stretches of the hip, hamstring, and inner thighs. Weight training on the ball kept his legs and ankles strong so he was able to make quick adjustments if his head and trunk jerked suddenly forward. Traditional weight-training methods that Art had used in the past worked lower and upper body separately. The goal with ballwork was to train the body as a unit, through a full range of motion, imitating the demands made by everyday life.

Around the time that he began ball classes Art started seeing a shiatsu practitioner who also did Rolfing. Rolfing is deep-tissue massage and manipulation that realigns the body by reorganizing the connective tissue surrounding the muscles. After a few sessions Art felt less stooped and his spine felt longer. He felt more alert and his wife claimed he no longer limped.

Posture: Staying in Line with Gravity

Finding a movement system or a practitioner that corrects alignment in the knees, pelvis, shoulders, or feet can change one's emotional outlook on life. Ida Rolf (1896–1979), inventor of the healing system Rolfing, believed that all behavior is expressed through the musculoskeletal system. "A man crying the blues is in reality bewailing his structural limitations and failures," she wrote. Unless a person's physical situation is changed, the emotional reality remains.

Without the proper foundation, how can one navigate through life never mind lift weights or add resistance to the body? When the chest muscles are concaved and shoulders are pulling forward, the effects are felt in the head, hips, knees, and feet. The opposite posture, what's commonly known as the military stance, with shoulders jerked back and chest lifted, locks the upper back. Weak abdominals can cause the pelvis to tilt so that the low-back curve is increased. On the other hand, short hamstring muscles cause the pelvis to tilt in the other direction, flattening the lumbar spine. Lack of equilibrium between muscles at the front of the hip and trunk and those at the back cause pain and problems in the whole body and can hamper proper breathing.

According to somatics pioneer Thomas Hanna, our sensorimotor system responds to daily strains and demands with specific muscle reflexes. The "red-light reflex" is a protective response to perceived fear. As the body withdraws from danger—or from stress, as the case may be—the abdominals tighten, the spine flexes inward, and the shoulders slump. The opposite response, the

Postural Assessment

*t*he skeleton is the framework of the body. When the body is correctly aligned, as shown in the drawing here, the plumb line is a line of reference around which the bones of the skeleton stack up. Ideally the plumb line should pass midway through the lobe of the ear and the joints of the shoulder, hip, knee, and ankle.

Very few people have ideal posture, though. When the ear lobes sit forward of the plumb line the alignment of the upper body is affected; this posture creates tension in the back of the neck. When the pelvis sits forward of the plumb line there is a problem with weight distribution in the knees and feet. Another common postural problem is the pelvis being tilted too far forward or too far back; both of these positions affect the hips and low back.

The pelvis in this drawing is in neutral: the front of the hipbones and the pubic bone line up in the same plane; the hipbones are not tilted too far forward or too far back.

When we retrain postural habits we try to work in neutral position and balance the three natural curves of the body. To find your vertical plumb line, make the following postural explorations.

- Stand in front of a mirror and if possible get someone to help assess you. Look at your ankles. Is the inside arch of your foot rolling in or out? Is the weight equally distributed between both feet? Perhaps one foot is "toeing" outward. If so, this is not just happening in the ankle; it is likely also happening higher up in the hip and pelvis. When you stand on your feet or sit on the ball are you able to feel the tripod position of the feet—base of big toe, base of little toe, and heel? When you stand are your knees rolling in (a knock-kneed position) or bowing out? Are they locked in place?

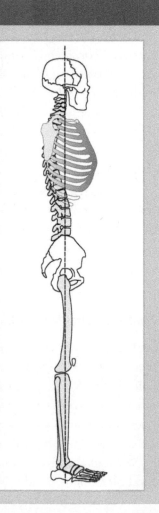

"green-light reflex," is triggered by the onslaught of daily responsibilities and chores, creating a chronic contracting of the back that leads to backache and stiffness. Hanna sees these two adaptive reflexes as having a profound effect on standing, walking posture, and aging.

Uncovering a New Neutral Spine

According to Mabel E. Todd, a pioneer writer in the field of body mechanics, old age is not gauged chronologically: "One becomes old when fixities of habits are established—set permanently—when the formation of new habits is no longer welcome." Happily, the position of our spines can alter as restrictions in our bodies ease.

The spine has four natural curves, the most important being the movable ones: the slightly concave curve of the cervical spine (the neck), the slightly convex curve of the upper back, and the concave curve of the lower back. There is a fourth, fixed curve in the sacrum, the triangular bone at the base of the spine. These curves in the spine are essential: in conjunction with the

Postural Assessment (continued)

- Is one side of the pelvis higher than the other? Get someone to check the most prominent bony surface of your pelvis—your hipbones. Are they horizontal?

- What about your sitz bones on the bottom of your pelvis? Sit on a hard chair. Is your weight on one sitz bone more than the other?

- Stand up again and look from the side as well as the front. Is your belly protruding? Is there an exaggerated curve in the low back? Or do you have a swayback posture, another common alignment problem caused by a pelvis that has moved forward of where it should be, resulting in a slumped appearance? Remember, the goal is not to flatten the back or create an exaggerated curve in the lower back, upper back, or neck. The goal is to preserve the natural curves of the spine without overtilting or tucking the pelvis.

- Now move up to the shoulders. Is one shoulder higher than the other? Do the collarbones roll for-

ward? Or are the shoulders pulled rigidly back, creating tension in the neck and upper back?

- What about your head? Neck pain and headaches are common ailments. Deep and superficial muscles of the neck work together to support the skull. If the neck vertebrae are not correctly aligned they can put pressure on important arteries that weave through the neck bones to the head. The head, neck, and shoulders function together: problems in one area will have a ripple effect into related structures.

- Ask someone to look at you from the side to judge where your head sits in relationship to your shoulders. Is the head protruding forward? Is your chin jutting upward? The head, which weighs twelve to sixteen pounds, should balance squarely and with minimal effort, with your ears positioned above your shoulders. Remember that the skull extends into the space behind you as well as the space in front of you.

proprioception

Proprioception is the sensory feedback that informs your body where it is in space. When your foot is about to step down on a stair, proprioceptors gather information about position and speed of the body and position and steepness of the step and send this data quickly to the brain. For the foot to find the step safely, clear information is necessary. If the receptors cease to give information to your brain you will have trouble maneuvering, as when your foot falls asleep and there is no information coming from the nerves. Have your vision checked regularly. Alertness and clear vision help the brain know where the body is in space and will make the difference between stepping in a hole or navigating around it.

Incoming proprioceptive stimuli can be manipulated by closing or opening your eyes and by wearing shoes or not. *The Swiss Ball* author and physical therapist, Beate Carrière, notes that sleeve-type braces improve proprioception. She believes this may be the reason that patients like to wrap a sprain or wear sleeve-type support for a long time following an injury.

gel-filled vertebral discs, they act as shock absorbers. The position of the spine with its natural curves in place is called neutral spine. When we retrain postural habits we are not trying to eliminate these natural curves, nor are we trying to exaggerate them. The goal is to balance these curves.

Time is needed to address the limitations of the body—time and a great deal of diligence. At first, being out of alignment feels "normal" for many people. Over the years the body aligns itself according to the demands made on it; new suggestions and organization feel wrong. The correct stretches and strengthening exercises are needed to create balance in muscle tone and length. Some students may need deeper bodywork to integrate and reestablish structure and ensure neuromuscular signals are flowing freely. Bit by bit, working over time, compensations are adjusted and a new neutral spine is uncovered.

Strength Training and Balance

When *Strong Women, Strong Bones* author Miriam E. Nelson completed her famed Tufts University study on strength training and postmenopausal women, an unexpected result emerged. It was discovered that strength training of the upper and lower body significantly improves balance. Her volunteers were middle-aged women. She found there to be an average 8 percent balance decline in women who did not strength train. On the other hand, the women in her strength training group showed an average 14 percent gain in balance scores. Her work reflects the findings in a 1997 New Zealand study that demonstrated a 53 percent reduction in falls in elderly women who did strength training and balance exercises.

Many coaches, trainers, and physical therapists now incorporate balance exercises into their strength-training programs. But it is helpful to know that strength training itself builds good balance. The stronger the legs, ankles, and calves, the quicker the muscles will contract to counteract against movement that pulls your body off equilibrium.

Strength training with balls requires even more balance and coordination than standard weight training. And the instability of the ball improves proprioception, the sensory feedback loop that informs your body of its position in space. Surprise and unpredictibility associated with the ball challenges the nervous system. Receptors give faster information to the brain. Quick reaction time prevents falls and stumbles.

As you approach the footwork and the balance tests included in this chapter, remember it is not only the feet that are working to keep you aligned and balanced. The small stabilizing muscles of the body make constant, slight adjustments to keep the body erect. A bodybuilder may be able to lift

350 pounds but will be knocked off center if the core and other stabilizers are weak. In the footwork we are not only working the lower body; we're working the whole body as a unit. Even the position of the head affects the body's overall balance.

The Footwork

Ida Rolf referred to the feet as "tattletales" because of how much they give away about imbalances higher up in the body. Before I started using the ball I taught traditional Pilates mat classes, where participants only got up and on their feet at the end of the hour for the final exercise. As the beginners stood up to do Roll Down the Wall or intermediate students went into the Pilates push-up, I could barely conceal my shock. Feet splayed open; ankles rolled inward; knees locked; and hips, shoulders, and head were misaligned. All the benefits of the previous hour dissolved in three seconds. I felt helpless to address the problems I saw in front of me.

The feet tell the story of how people step, use their weight, and keep their balance. The foot is an intricate collection of small bones strung together with muscles, tendons, and ligaments. If the foot were rigid like a block of cement it would just bang and chip as it touched the ground, but instead the foot is designed to absorb shock. Think of the foot as a three-dimensional pyramid. The arches work like little suspension bridges and affect all the structures from the ankles upward. When you are standing up or sitting on the ball, focus your attention often on your feet (without actually looking down to observe them). Think of your foot like a three-dimensional tripod—the key bases of support being the base of the big toe, the base of the little toe, and the heel. Distribute your weight equally between these three bases and between both feet.

The following exercises are designed to build balance, bring the body back into alignment, and strengthen the muscles of the feet, ankles, buttocks, legs, and thighs. This includes strengthening the muscles that keep your knee tracking correctly over your second toe. Take care that the knee lines up with the ankle and swings forward and backward like a hinge on a door. Knee and ankle joints are hinge joints and are not constructed for much rotation. Work in good foot-knee alignment so as not to weaken the hinge.

The balance tests in the check-in may surprise you. Try them again in two weeks and see if you notice a difference. Don't skip through the postural check-in. Answer all the questions and get someone else to assess you if possible.

The Footwork Exercises

This movement series is performed against a wall. Make sure you place your feet far enough away from the wall so that when you bend the legs the knees don't jut out over the toes. Keep neutral pelvis and let the tailbone feel heavy; be careful that the tailbone does not roll back around the ball. Remember that the goal is to preserve the natural curves of the spine without overtilting or tucking the pelvis.

Relax your shoulders and gaze straight ahead. Bring special attention to the knees, making sure the center of the kneecap tracks properly over the second toe. Avoid locking the knees back into the legs when you straighten; pull up the muscles above the knee to keep the kneecap tracking properly. Placing a small ball between your knees may help align your legs; a gentle squeeze of the ball will target the adductors, the muscles that bring the legs together.

Stand Up: Are Your Feet a Reliable Base or Not?

*i*f your ankles are weak or a part of your foot is unbalanced, a chain reaction sets in. The knee rolls in, the inside arch of the foot collapses, and the body adapts by tightening up. Before you know it the ligaments of the foot, ankle, and knee have taken on a whole new shape. You experience pains in your heels or arches and notice the actual shape of the foot is changing as bunions build up and/or toes cross over. When feet don't do their jobs properly, providing comfort and shock absorption such as they are designed for, shin splints, fallen arches, plantar fasciitis, stress fractures, and other physical disturbances result.

Think of your foot as a three-dimensional

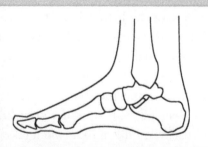

tripod, the key bases of support being the base of the big toe, the base of the little toe, and the heel. Spread the weight equally between these three bases, remembering that the foot has three primary arches: the inner arch, the outer arch, and the arch across the front of the foot. It is the arches, stabilized by muscles in the leg and the foot, that provide the spring that allows the foot to spread out and bounce back.

Working with Pilates movement in bare feet is a great way to regain a connection with gravity. Shoes stop your sensory nerves from feeling the ground and providing proprioceptive feedback. If you find your feet slipping, work on a sticky yoga mat.

For variety and challenge, hold weights or wrap a resistance band across the bottom of the feet. When using the band keep the thumbs upward and the wrists strong (not bent at the crease), slowly pull up the band as you bend the knees. Do not add weights or bands until you are able to coordinate all the movements and work in good patterns.

Purpose To strengthen legs, buttocks, ankles, and muscles of the thighs. Weights and resistance bands build the upper arms: in side lift, they build the deltoids and rotator cuff; in front lift, the lats and deltoids; in biceps curls, they work the biceps.

Watchpoints • Don't bend the knees too much; keep the center of the kneecap aligned over the second toe and avoid rolling the ankles in or out. • Maintain the navel-to-spine connection. • In movement 2 be sure that you are turning out or in from the hip sockets and not the feet. In movement 5, ensure that the band is secure under your feet so that it does not snap out. • Keep the thumbs upward and the wrists strong. • Review band safety precautions on page 53.

starting position

Place your ball against the wall and roll the body so that the ball is in the curve at the lower back. Press your weight back into the ball without leaning too far back. Stand with the heels approximately 20 to 28 inches from the wall. Your feet should be hip-distance apart. If desired, place a small ball between the knees for movements 1 and 3. Hands are relaxed at your side; knees are aligned over the feet.

movement 1: parallel feet

1. Feet are hip-distance apart and parallel **(fig. 4.1)**. Exhale to bend the knees, keeping

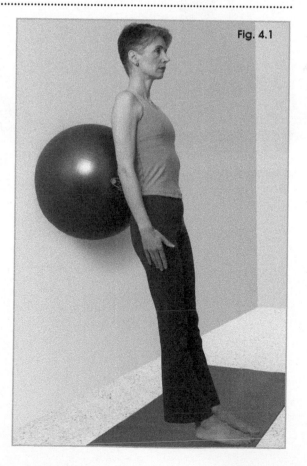

Fig. 4.1

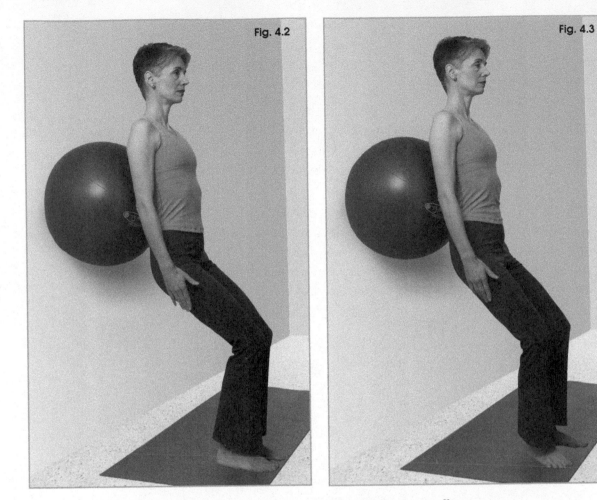

Fig. 4.2

Fig. 4.3

the heels down **(fig. 4.2)**.
2. Inhale to straighten the legs. Repeat six to eight times.

movement 2: small turnout

1. Begin with heels together, legs slightly turned out and toes in a V shape. Exhale to bend the knees, keeping the heels on the floor **(fig. 4.3)**.
2. Inhale to straighten the legs. Repeat six to eight times.

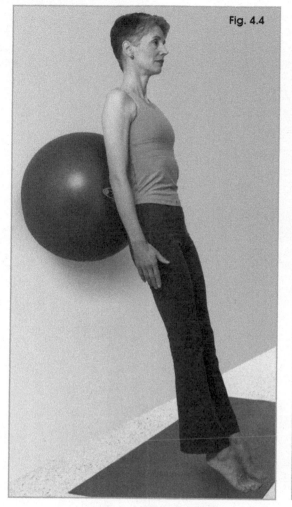

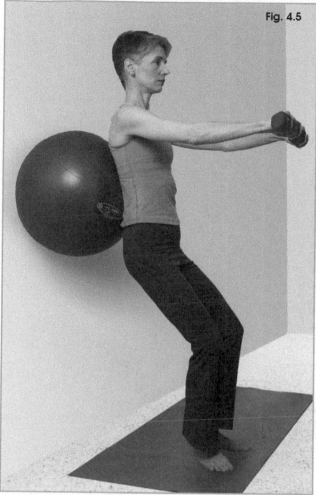

movement 3: calf raises

1. Set the feet back to parallel. Inhale to lift up on high half-toe **(fig. 4.4)**.
2. Exhale to put the heels down.
3. Inhale to lift the heels. Exhale to lower.
4. Repeat six to eight times.

movement 4: add weights

1. Hold in your hands 1-, 2-, or 3-pound weights. As you bend knees in either parallel or turnout position, lift your arms to the side or front **(fig. 4.5)**. Ensure that the arms do not lift above shoulder level.
2. Repeat six to eight times.

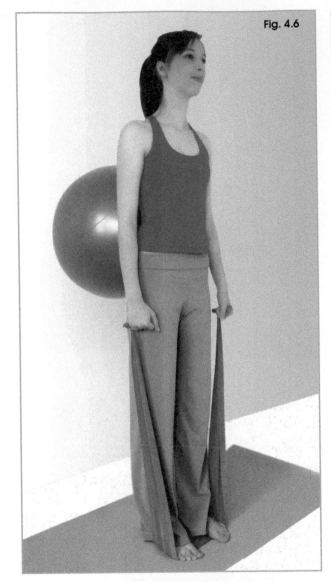

Fig. 4.6

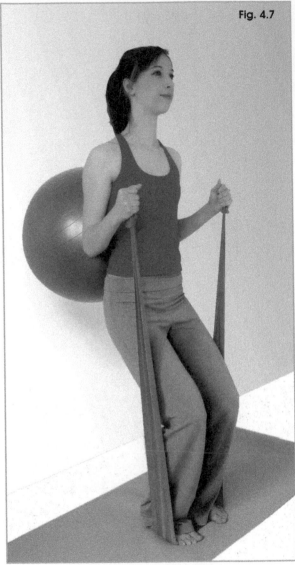

Fig. 4.7

movement 5: resistance band bicep curls

1. Place the band widely across the floor and stand on it. Feet are parallel and hip-distance apart **(fig. 4.6)**.

2. On the exhalation, in one movement bend the knees to lower your body and bend the elbows to pull up on the band. The thumbs face upward and the wrists are strong **(fig. 4.7)**.

3. Inhale to straighten the legs and the elbows, lowering the arms but keeping the band taut. Repeat six to eight times.

Squats with and without Weights

In this movement series you should feel an oppositional stretch in the body; as you bend the knees feel the sensation of the head elongating upward, as if the crown of the head is attached to a string. As you ground the feet into the mat, the upper body naturally lengthens and releases upward—you will experience a stretch in the spine that can be felt long after you finish the exercise. You can add 1-, 2-, or 3-pound weights for more resistance.

Purpose To strengthen the quadriceps, including the muscles above the knee responsible for keeping it tracking correctly. To strengthen the gluteals and the small external rotators of the thigh. Weights add challenge to the upper body.

Watchpoints • Make sure your kneecaps are tracking over the second toe and not rolling inward. • Avoid deep bends; work in your pain-free range.

starting position

Place your ball against the wall and roll the body so that the ball is in the curve at the low back. Press your weight back into the ball but do not collapse into it. Stand with the heels approximately 20 to 28 inches from the wall.

movement 1: wide squat with bicep curls

1. Begin with feet wider than shoulder-distance apart and slightly turned out **(fig. 4.8)**.

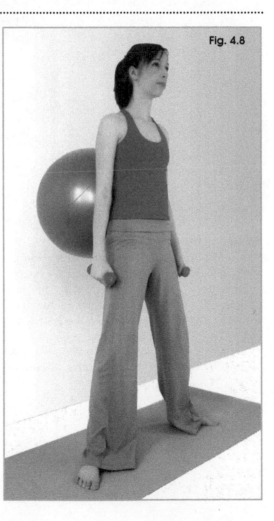

Fig. 4.8

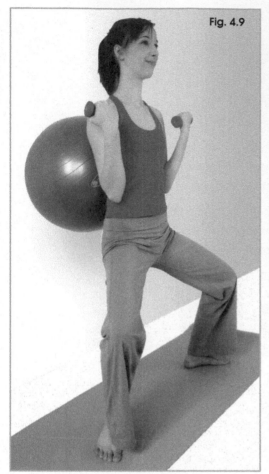

Fig. 4.9

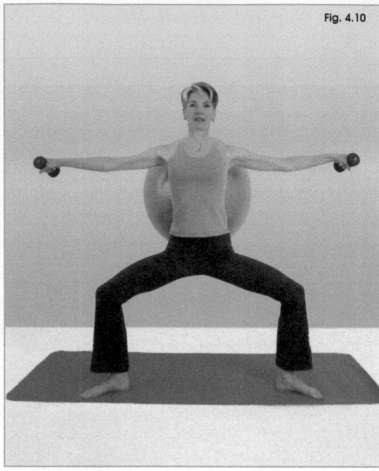

Fig. 4.10

2. Exhale to bend the knees and curl the forearms, keeping the long bones of the upper arm in place **(fig. 4.9)**. The center of the kneecap should be aligned over the second toe.
3. Inhale to straighten the legs. Repeat six to eight times.

movement 2: side raises

1. Begin with feet wider than shoulder-distance apart and slightly turned out.
2. Exhale to bend the knees and lift the arms straight up from the sides to shoulder height. The palms face downward **(fig. 4.10)**.
3. Inhale to straighten the legs and lower the arms. Repeat six to eight times.

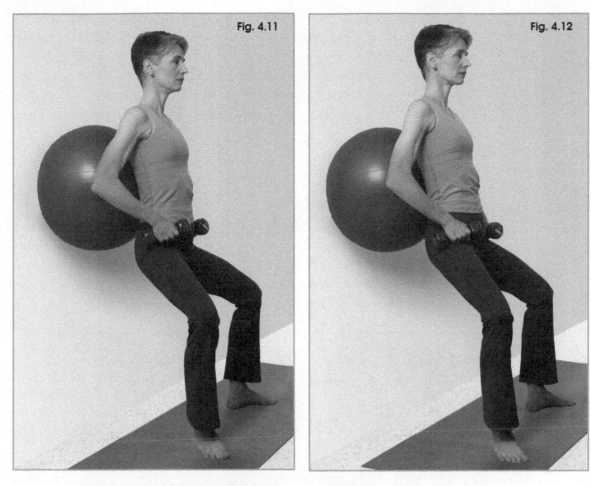

Fig. 4.11

Fig. 4.12

movement 3: isolate the belly of the muscle (intermediate)

1. Set your weights on your thighs to add extra challenge. Exhale to bend the knees, keeping the heels down **(fig. 4.11)**.

2. Inhale to come up two inches **(fig. 4.12)**.

3. Exhale deeper in the squat. Inhale to come up only two inches.

4. Repeat six to eight times, emphasizing the down position.

Single-Leg Footwork and Lunges

Working on one leg really tests your balance as well as builds strength in the quadriceps, gluteals, and ankles. Facing the wall, work one leg and then the other, raising up on a high half-toe or bending the knee, all the while keeping your balance on one leg. For movement 3, single-leg lunge, place the ball in a corner or use a cane for assistance—this is a very challenging exercise and it is easy to lose your balance. Keep your back straight and your chest lifted as you bend and straighten the knee. Avoid twisting the knee: the center of the kneecap needs to stay aligned over the second toe to ensure proper structure. Make sure that the knee does not poke out over the foot. Take care coming out of single-leg lunge that you don't strain your back leg as you swing it through. Use a smaller ball if necessary so the back leg is not lifted too high.

Purpose To work the quadriceps, gluteals, and hamstrings; strengthen the hips; and balance the muscles around the buttocks and legs. Notice that in movement 3 the hip flexors and deep thigh muscle is stretched in the back leg when the leg is up on the ball.

Watchpoints • Keep the upper body straight and the shoulders and hips facing forward. • Keep the tailbone heavy and the pelvis in neutral. • In movement 3 be sure that your front foot is far enough away from the wall so that when you bend the knee the lower leg remains vertical and is not too far forward over the toes. • If you have knee problems avoid movement 3.

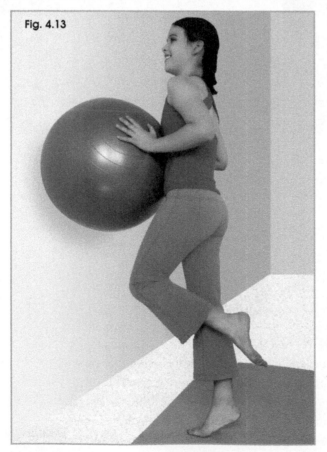

Fig. 4.13

starting position

Place the ball against the wall and face the ball. Place your hands on the ball.

movement 1: single-leg footwork, high half-toe

1. Feet are hip-distance apart and parallel. Lift the left foot off the mat and lift the right heel up to high half-toe position **(fig. 4.13)**.
2. Exhale to set the right heel back on the mat.
3. Inhale to lift the right heel. Repeat six to eight times and switch sides.

movement 2: single-leg footwork, bend and stretch

1. Feet are hip-distance apart and parallel. As above, lift the left foot off the mat.
2. Exhale to bend the right knee, keeping the heel down.
3. Inhale to straighten the right leg.
4. Repeat six to eight times and switch sides.

movement 3: single-leg lunge (intermediate)

1. Place the ball in a corner for stability. Place the right leg back up on the ball, using the wall to balance you. The tops of your toes should be on the top side of the ball. Hop out far enough away from the corner so that when you bend the knee your front toe does not poke over your knee. Keep the toes of both feet pointing directly forward **(fig. 4.14)**. If necessary, use a cane for balance.

2. On the exhale, and keeping the torso straight, bend your forward knee. Your back leg is straight behind you, toes pointing forward. Keep your body upright **(fig. 4.15)**.

3. Inhale to straighten the knee.

4. Repeat six to eight times and switch sides.

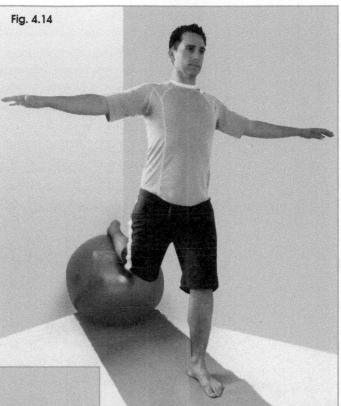

Fig. 4.14

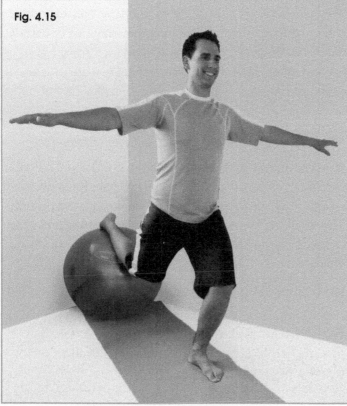

Fig. 4.15

Each of us has inherited structural tendencies and molded body shapes for ourselves and these cannot be changed overnight. You may need to work one-on-one with a practitioner who specializes in postural realignment or deep-tissue work to bring your body back into balance. The focus of the next chapter is on strengthening the abdominal core as well as the floor of the pelvis. This will not only trim the waistline but ensure better posture and alignment. A strong core brings support to the spine and properly prepares the body for adding resistance.

As you worked through the previous exercises you may have noticed that your balance is not as good as you thought it was. The following check-in will help test your balance and determine whether your posture is sound.

Check-In: Balance Tests and Postural Assessment

Poor balance and slow reactions can cause falls. For Test 1, some people whose balance is impaired may want to begin by sitting on a stable surface such as a chair or a Physio Roll, a peanut-shaped ball that rolls only in one direction (the ball shown in these instructions). You may need to have a steady surface nearby to hold on to. Start by sitting in the center of the ball, feet parallel and hip-distance apart. Press your hands against the side of the ball to stabilize your core before you lift one foot. Then try balancing on one foot or narrowing your base of support. Closing your eyes ups the balance stakes, as your vision tells your brain important information about where you are in space. If you feel unsteady or dizzy during any of the tests, stop immediately.

Test 1: Sitting

Sitting on the ball is an excellent method for improving posture and balance. Make sure there is enough space between the legs and the ball. Keep the head aligned and the chin horizontal; visualize a string pulling you upward from the crown of the head. The shoulders are relaxed as you lengthen through the tops of the ears. Keep your hands on the ball to stabilize the core; taking your hands away increases the challenge.

Purpose To sit in good neutral spine and to test your balance.

Watchpoints • Do not lose optimal posture or neutral spine as you close your eyes or adjust your feet. • Keep the chin horizontal, eyes level. • Keep your hands on the ball; press the hands gently into the side of the ball to stabilize your core. • Do not hold your breath.

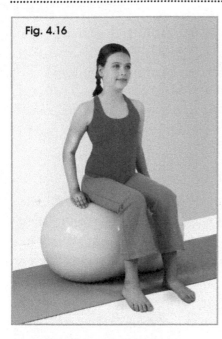

Fig. 4.16

Fig. 4.17

Fig. 4.18

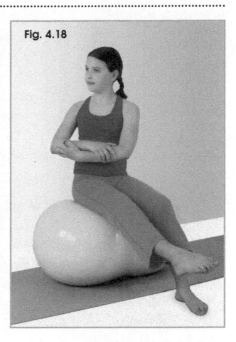

starting position

Make sure you're sitting on the center of your ball. Feet are parallel and planted hip-distance apart.

movement 1: open eyes

Sit tall and breathe naturally **(fig. 4.16)**.

movement 2: close eyes

Sit tall and breathe naturally. Close your eyes and hold your position.

movement 3: lift foot

1. Lift one foot two inches above the ground and hold **(fig. 4.17)**, or place the foot on a small soggy ball and hold. Breathe naturally.
2. Repeat on the other side. Increase "hold" time as you can.

movement 4: lift leg with rotation

1. Lift one leg two inches above the ground and hold. On the inhalation, rotate the body in the direction of the raised leg **(fig. 4.18)**.
2. Exhale to return to center.
3. Inhale to place the foot back on mat.
4. Exhale to lift the opposite leg and inhale to rotate the body in the opposite direction. Repeat from side to side.

movement 5: narrow the base of support

Narrow your feet so that your ankles and knees are touching. Or place both feet on a small ball **(fig. 4.19)**. Sit tall and breathe naturally. Increase "hold" time if possible.

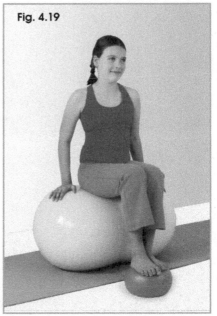

Fig. 4.19

keeping upright: righting and tilting reflexes

Working on a mobile ball is believed to improve the speed of righting and tilting reflexes. These reflexes, developed soon after we are born, underlie movement patterns and help the body interact with gravity.

Righting reflexes are the reactions used to bring the head in line with the spine and to keep our bodies upright against gravity when the body is on a stationary surface. Tilting reflexes, sometimes called equilibrium responses, maintain balance when your center of gravity is shifted. For example as you walk on a moving sidewalk at an airport your tilting reflexes work to adjust your center of balance and keep your head aligned.

A person with good righting and tilting reflexes will easily make the split-second adjustments necessary to remain upright in everyday experiences. Many falls could be avoided by improving your righting and tilting reflexes.

Test 2: Standing

The strength of your core will help you stay upright when balancing on one leg. If you're working specifically on improving your balance, try these moves each day, holding them longer each time. Close your eyes for an extra challenge and ask someone to time you to see how long you can stand with your eyes closed or on one foot. Remember to activate the navel-to-spine connection to keep the stabilizers strong. If you feel unsteady or dizzy during any of the tests, stop immediately.

Purpose To challenge balance and test the deep stabilizers.

Watchpoints • Do not rush in or out of the balances. • Keep your shoulders relaxed. • Keep the pelvis in neutral, tailbone down. • Ensure that the standing leg is always slightly bent so that you are not pressing the knee back into hyperextension. • Make sure the area around you is clear in case you lose your balance.

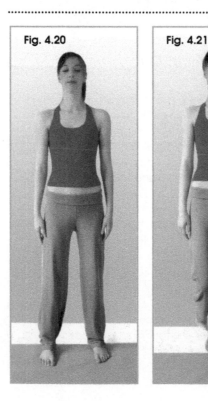

Fig. 4.20   Fig. 4.21

movement 1: standing with closed eyes

1. Stand on two legs with your weight equally distributed. Close your eyes **(fig. 4.20)**.
2. Breathing naturally, hold this position for 20 to 30 seconds.

movement 2: single leg

1. Open your eyes. Ground your left foot into the mat and shift the weight to that foot as you lift the right foot **(fig. 4.21)**. Focus on a point on the wall and hold for 20 seconds.
2. Breathe smoothly. Repeat on the other side. Over time increase the "hold" time if possible.

If you take your balance for granted you may not do so after trying these tests. Do them alone, with friends, or with your children—if young people practice balance exercises it will keep them physically "sharp" for later years, when a chronic fear of falling can lead to a drastic reduction in activities. Repeat the balance tests often and time yourself to see if you can increase your "hold" time.

Working out with an unstable ball or standing on one foot not only challenges your balance but also trains your nervous system. It works like this: moving or sitting on the ball or being on one foot destabilizes your body. The sensory nerves, perceiving that you are off-kilter, send rapid messages to your brain and spinal cord. The brain then quickly instructs the muscles to make the adjustments necessary to keep you from falling. Forcing your nervous system to confront unfamiliar and ever-changing circumstances improves your reaction time. Good reaction time ensures that you possess the balance skills to confidently and safely move through your world.

5

The Abdominals:
The Powerhouse
to Strength

Owie, owie, that hurts.

—Cindy

Cindy's Story: Activating the Elevator at the Base
of the Powerhouse

Cindy, forty-seven, had consulted her doctor because of abnormally heavy menstrual periods. Two weeks later, concerned by something suspicious that had turned up in the test, the doctor was explaining the procedure for an abdominal hysterectomy, surgery by means of an incision through the layers of skin and fascia that line the abdomen. She tried to reassure Cindy that this was a routine procedure and that more than one women in four will have a hysterectomy by the time she reaches sixty. Yet Cindy knew that no surgery is to be taken lightly. Cindy's sister, who gave birth via cesarean section a decade earlier, felt that she still could not make her abdominal muscles work properly.

Cindy and I worked together two months after the operation and her spirits were good. Thankfully the earlier reports of tissue "pathology" turned out to be nonmalignant irregularities in the uterus and no more follow-up operations or treatments were necessary. Yet for Cindy it still felt as though a brick was lodged in her belly. She was very guarded in her movements. Moreover, she felt soreness in her neck, shoulders, and other parts of her body as these muscles overworked in place of her abdominals. For the first month she couldn't even sit up tall in a straight-back chair. "I'll never take my abs for granted again," she told me.

When the deep abdominals are properly contracted, the abdominal wall will narrow by wrapping around the low back like a corset. In the weeks following the operation Cindy couldn't believe that she would ever feel this "corseting" effect again. Instead, Cindy's abdomen felt domed and bloated. I decided to focus on another approach—to work through the pelvic floor to help Cindy rediscover power in her core.

Located on the bottom of the pelvis, the pelvic floor is the sling of muscles and ligaments that extends from the tailbone and sitz bones underneath the pelvis to the pubic bone in front. These muscles are used to control the flow of urine and feces; they provide support to the organs lying within the bony home of the pelvis. The pelvic-floor muscles are seen by more and more Pilates practitioners as an important part of the powerhouse, the abdominal core of the body. A strong pelvic floor is as important for men as it is for women because of how the pelvic floor neurologically connects through the nervous system to the deep abdominals.

Without allowing the tailbone to lift off the mat or the buttocks muscles to engage, I wanted Cindy to feel the pelvic-floor muscles—and only the pelvic-floor muscles—gently squeeze together. "Imagine," I told her, "the pelvic floor as an elevator drawing upward from floor to floor. Now pretend you have an extremely full bladder and tighten these muscles to hold back the flow of urine while you search for a bathroom."

Over the weeks that followed Cindy used the pelvic floor to help fire the deep abdominals. She placed her fingertips one inch in from her hipbones, in the direction of the pubic bone, and pressed in gently but deeply to feel for herself the powerhouse in action. I reminded her that she should feel a continual subtle tension in her fingertips as the deep abdominals are activated. Touch adds vital information to the brain's ability to sense the connection.

The Powerhouse: A Three-Dimensional Cylinder

Joseph Pilates regarded the abdominal area, in conjunction with the low back, as the "girdle of strength"—the powerhouse of the body. The stronger the girdle of strength, the more powerful and efficient the movement. Following Pilates' teachings, before each Pilates exercise we recruit the deep muscles of the low back and abdomen to keep the midsection stable before engaging in movements of the arms and legs.

The superficial and deep abdominal muscles work with the spinal muscles to make up the powerhouse. The superficial rectus abdominis runs down the front of the abdomen and is responsible for flexing the long trunk by pulling the ribs toward the pelvis. On the back of the spine is the erector spinae; these muscles, close to the surface of the body, make powerful movements such as arching of the back. The external and internal obliques are sheets of muscles that crisscross the body. They are responsible for sidebending and twisting and play a secondary role in stabilization.

It is the small muscles, the ones that are more internal to the body, that are the most important in stabilizing the powerhouse. Overlooked in some training, their function is to stabilize the low back and pelvis and keep this region free from pain. The Australian authorities on spinal stabilization—Carolyn Richardson, Gwendolen Jull, Paul Hodges, and Julie Hides—describe the deep stabilizing muscles of the abdomen and low back as a three-dimensional cylinder. On the front and side of the cylinder is the transversus abdominis, a deep muscle that wraps horizontally around the spine like a corset. This muscle has attracted a lot of attention lately because of its association with the prevention of low-back pain. Another important player is the zipper on the back of the corset: multifidus—small, deep bundles that pass from vertebra to verterbra. Stuart McGill, Ph.D., a leading expert on low-back disorders, believes that all of the trunk muscles play some role in stabilization, but multifidus and part of quadratus lumborum have been identified as key back stabilizers. Next is the base of the cylinder: the pelvic floor, the hammock of muscles that provides support for the inner organs. Finally, there is the lid of the cylinder: the dome-shaped breathing muscle, the diaphragm.

The stability of the low back depends on all the muscles of the powerhouse working together to transform the abdomen and spine into a strong cylinder of support.

Crunches Versus Curls

Traditional abdominal conditioning is often approached as a series of swift, vigorous sit-ups, or "crunches." Students pin their feet under a sofa or under their trainer's hands and curl rapidly forward, coming up as high as possible. Many repetitions with rapid speed can pull neck muscles, hunch shoulders, and compress the low back. In a Pilates curl, as opposed to traditional crunches or situps, we maintain the pelvis in neutral. This means that when you curl the body up you are not deliberately flattening the low back onto the mat.

Another limitation of traditional sit-ups is that they drill the body in one fixed direction and are designed to mainly strengthen the superficial rectus abdominis and parts of the psoas. Emphasizing rectus training creates short and thick abdominal muscles and a rib cage that is pulled too close to the pelvis, distorting the body. The psoas, another long, strong muscle, originates on the bony parts of the vertebrae of the lower spine, crosses the front of the

How to Work the Abdominals After Childbirth

*a*fter a vaginal birth, focus on toning and shortening the abdominals, not on elongating them, as they have already been stretched to their limit. Avoid large, challenging exercises such as lifting the legs high in the air; instead, keep limbs close to the body. The pelvic floor may be stretched or torn during childbirth, so to eliminate low-back pain and other problems, perform the pelvic floor exercises shown on pages 42, 81, and 82. To prevent pulling on the scar after a cesarean delivery, no exercise and limited movement for five to eight days are recommended. Six weeks after a cesarean you can begin your exercise routine, but resume exercise gradually after being given the "all clear" by your health care practitioner.

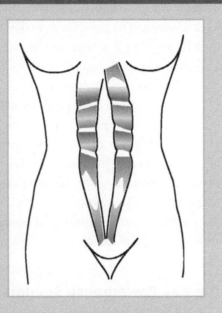

Sometimes diastasis recti (shown in diagram) occurs during pregnancy or following birth. This is the separation of the rectus abdominal muscles around the navel and is less common with women who have strong abs before pregnancy. You will notice a vertical bulge in the middle of your abdomen. Strenuous exercise must be avoided until the diastasis recti is corrected. Specialized exercises such as Navel-to-Spine, pelvic tilts on the hands and knees, and small ab curls with the arms hugged around the body will decrease the width of the separation. If necessary, work with a therapist to correct the problem.

pelvis, and attaches at the top of the inner thighbone. Its function is to flex the hip, bringing the leg closer to the trunk; because the psoas is often a strong, overtrained muscle it can rush to the aid of the abdominals in traditional conditioning exercises.

The goal in a Pilates approach to abdominal strengthening is to lengthen and integrate the psoas into the abdominal work. In some cases this means beginning with stretching the psoas and strengthening the abdominals. Tight hip flexors and weak abdominals can cause problems in the low back, the pelvis, or even the upper back. Then we focus on integrating the psoas into the abdominal work. We do this by focusing on the eccentric or lengthening contraction of both the psoas and the rectus abdominis. An eccentric contraction is when the muscle lengthens under load in a controlled way. In fact, the lengthening contraction, in which you use the muscles as brakes as you elongate the body carefully back into its starting position on the ball or mat, is more work for the muscles. Utilizing the full range of motion is a much more balanced way to strengthen the abdominals.

The curl-up is a much smaller movement than a traditional sit-up. With the curl-up we keep the pelvis stable and maintain the natural curve in the low back, only flexing the upper body so that the shoulder blades just barely lift off the mat. The hands are loosely clasped at the base of the skull or stretched down the mat. In some cases you will hold the body in a position without movement, increasing the tension in the muscle without changing its length. This is called an isometric contraction, and it builds the endurance of the muscles.

The Key Powerhouse Builders

The exercises in this chapter are the key powerhouse builders from the Pilates repertoire. I have added large and small balls to introduce greater challenge and resistance. The weight of the ball makes the abs work extra hard. These effective exercises are designed to increase the strength and endurance of the abdominal muscles and in some cases alleviate moderate low-back pain. Think of drawing in your lower abdomen, between the navel and the pubic bone, and remember that it is the exhalation that aids you in activating the deep abdominals. If you have a sore neck, leave your head on the mat or place your hands behind your neck to support it whenever you lift your head off the mat. See the box "Curling the Head off the Mat" on page 92.

Pelvic-Floor Elevator

A strong pelvic floor is as important for men as it is for women. Remember, the pelvis itself should not move and the gluteals should remain relaxed; only the muscles on the bottom of the pelvis will gently draw up and in as they tighten. Imagine that you have an extremely full bladder and are tightening these muscles to stop the flow of urine. Women may recognize the Pelvic Floor Elevator as a variation on a Kegel exercise.

Purpose To locate the pelvic floor and to keep tension in the muscles as you breathe naturally.

Watchpoints • Do not let the pelvis move or tilt—keep it in neutral. • Recruit the pelvic floor gently and evenly, front and back, and make sure the gluteals remain relaxed.

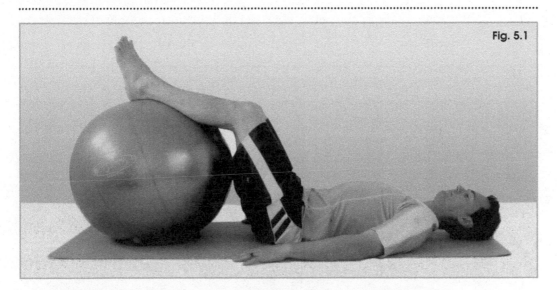

Fig. 5.1

starting position

Lie on your back. Place your feet hip-distance apart on the mat or relax them up on a ball. The head and shoulders are relaxed. The hands are stretched down the mat.

movement: pelvic-floor elevator

1. Take a couple of easy, relaxing breaths.
2. On the exhalation, gently draw the pelvic floor upward. Imagine an elevator ascending from the basement to the first floor. Do not squeeze the gluteals or lift the pelvis **(fig. 5.1)**.
3. Maintain the elevator on the first floor and hold the contraction for 3 to 5 seconds, breathing naturally.
4. On the exhalation, slowly draw the elevator from the first floor to the second floor. Hold the contraction for 3 to 5 seconds, breathing naturally.
5. Repeat this up to floor six. Then totally release, allowing the elevator to descend slowly to the basement.

Knee-Lift Stabilizing Exercise

Begin this classic stabilizing exercise on a mat and then try it on a slightly underinflated small ball. Remember to initiate from the hip, not the knee; use the drawing in and tightening of the pelvic floor to aid you in finding the deep abdominal connection. Then test the pelvic floor-transversus abdominis connection by placing your three middle fingertips one inch from the hipbones; press in gently but deeply. You should feel a continual subtle tension in your fingertips as the tranversus is activated.

In movements 2 and 3, nestle the small ball on the back of your pelvis (not in the low back). After mastering one leg at a time, hold both legs in the air in the tabletop position, a 90-degree angle of the knee. Take care to keep the abdominals contracted while you lift the second knee. The low back will gently imprint onto the small ball when both legs are up in the air.

Purpose To locate the pelvic floor and find the deep abdominal connection.

Watchpoints • Do not let the pelvis move or tilt. • If you no longer feel tension at your fingertips, use the modification and don't raise the knee so high. • It is more important to maintain the contraction than to lift the knee high.

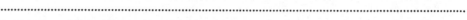

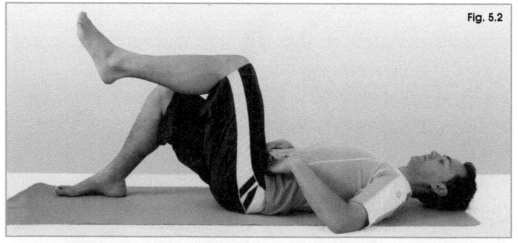

Fig. 5.2

starting position

Lie on your back. Place your feet hip-distance apart on the mat. Head and shoulders are relaxed. Place the tips of your three longest fingers one inch in from your hipbones and press in gently but deeply.

movement 1: knee-lift stabilizing exercise on mat

1. Take a couple of easy, relaxing breaths.
2. On the next exhalation draw in your lower abdomen, pull up the pelvic floor, and take a breath or two.
3. Then, keeping the abdominals and pelvic floor activated, on an exhalation lift the left knee to a tabletop position **(fig. 5.2)**. Can you feel the subtle pressure

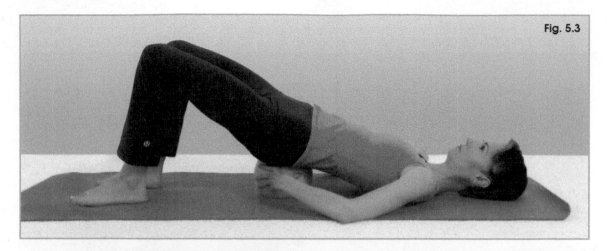

Fig. 5.3

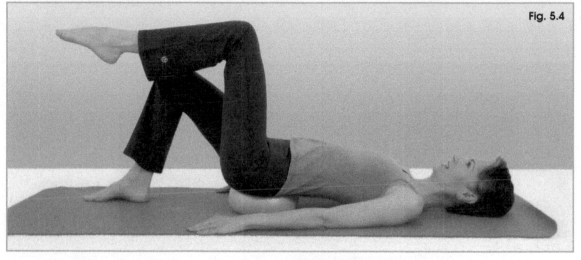

Fig. 5.4

on your fingertips as the pelvic-floor contraction activates the deep abdominals? You should feel the muscle flatten rather than bulge.

4. Inhale and stay. Exhale to return the left foot to the mat.

5. Repeat four times on each side, one leg at a time.

movement 2: knee-lift stabilizing exercise on small ball

1. Still lying on your back, feet on mat, lift up your pelvis and nestle a slightly deflated small ball under your hips. The small ball will rest under the pelvis, not in the low back **(fig. 5.3)**. Stretch your fingertips down the mat.

2. Exhale to draw in your lower abdomen, gently pull up the pelvic floor, and find the deep abdominal contraction.

3. Inhale to keep the contraction. Exhale to lift the left knee so that the leg is in tabletop position **(fig. 5.4)**. Control the movement with your abdominals and pelvic floor; do not think of initiating the movement from the quads or the hip flexors, the muscles at the front of the hip.

4. Inhale to lower the left foot slowly back onto the mat.

5. Exhale to lift the right knee to tabletop position.

6. Repeat four to six times, maintaining awareness of the abdominal connection.

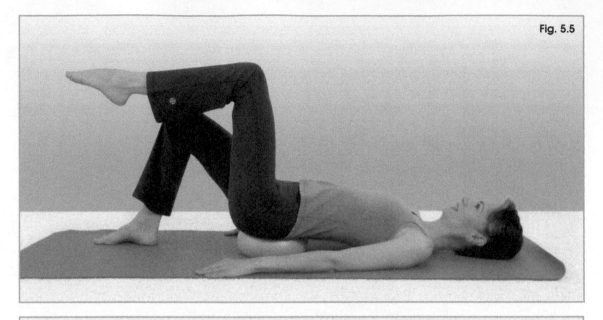

Fig. 5.5

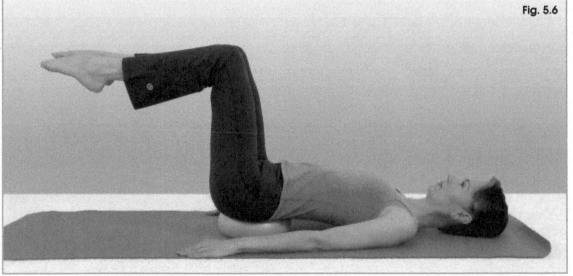

Fig. 5.6

movement 3: double-knee lift

1. With the small ball still resting under the pelvis, stretch your fingertips down the mat. Inhale to prepare.
2. Exhale to draw in your lower abdomen and gently pull up the pelvic floor.
3. Inhale to keep the contraction; exhale to maintain the contraction and lift the left leg to tabletop position **(fig. 5.5)**.

4. Inhale and stay to keep the contraction as you hold the left leg up.
5. Exhale to lift the right leg to join the left leg in the tabletop position. The legs will be slightly apart and the low back will imprint on the small ball **(fig. 5.6)**. Inhale and stay in tabletop legs.
6. Exhale to bring both feet slowly down to the mat, hip-distance apart.
7. Repeat six to eight times.

Abdominal Curls

In the previous exercise you learned to draw in and tighten the pelvic floor. Utilize this pelvic-floor–abdominal connection as you practice these curls. When the legs are placed up on the ball, maintain the legs in alignment and the pelvis in neutral. This means that when you curl the body up you are not deliberately flattening the low back onto the mat; instead, keep the low back in its natural curve. Make sure there is flexion in the upper back and that the abdominals, deep and superficial, are working—after all, this is not a neck stretch. Imagine you are gently drawing your navel away from the edge of your pants toward your spine.

Purpose To strengthen the abdominals.

Watchpoints • The pelvis stays in neutral and the tailbone does not lift as you curl the upper body upward. • Do not curl up too high: the shoulder blades just barely clear the mat. Make sure the head comes up immediately and the gaze is on your knees, not on the ceiling. • Do not pull on the neck; elbows are wide.

starting position

Lie on your back with the ball under your knees, knees in line with your hips; make sure your knees don't splay outward. Place your hands loosely at the base of the skull **(fig. 5.7)**.

movement 1: ab curls, legs on the ball

1. Inhale to prepare, keeping your head on the mat.
2. Exhale to draw the navel gently toward the spine and flex the upper body, lifting the head **(fig. 5.8)**.
3. Inhale and stay in this position. Keep the abdominals connected. Gently draw your navel away from the edge of your pants.
4. Exhale to return your head to the mat.
5. Repeat eight times in a slow and controlled manner.

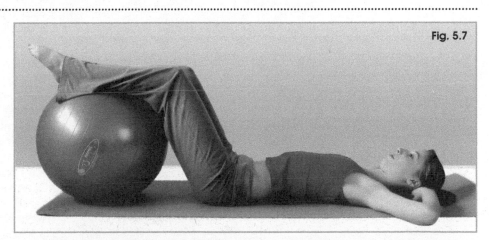
Fig. 5.7

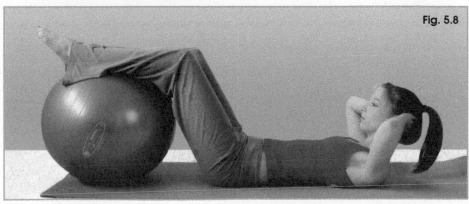
Fig. 5.8

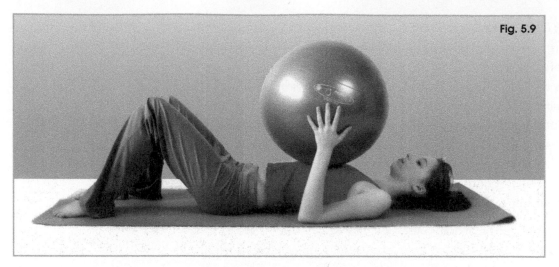

Fig. 5.9

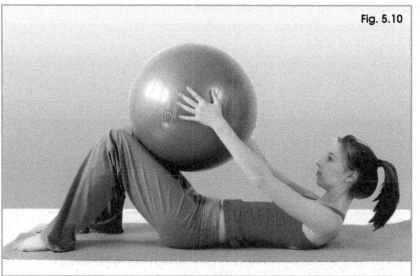

Fig. 5.10

movement 2: hold contraction

1. Begin in the same starting position. If desired, stretch your fingertips down the mat. Inhale to prepare.

2. Exhale to draw the navel toward the spine and flexing the upper body, lifting the head.

3. Inhale and stay, tightening your abdominals. Your gaze is on your knees, not the ceiling. Take two breaths, holding this isometric contraction for three seconds. Exhale to return the head to the mat.

4. Repeat eight times.

movement 3: ab curls, feet on mat

1. Pick the ball up between your feet, lift the ball into the air, and place it into your hands. Then set the ball on your rib cage, hands on the side of the ball **(fig. 5.9)**. Inhale to prepare; the chin is slightly dropped but keep your head on the mat.

2. Exhale to sink the navel toward the spine and lift the head, flexing the upper body and rolling the ball up the legs **(fig. 5.10)**. Don't hyperextend the elbows. Instead, keep the elbows slightly bent.

3. Inhale and stay in this position. Keep the abdominals connected, pelvis in neutral.

4. Exhale to return the head to the mat and the ball to the rib cage.

5. Repeat eight times in a slow and controlled manner. If desired, hold the contraction for three seconds as in movement 2 but do not hold your breath.

The Roll-up

This exercise can be done with a small or large ball in the hands, but ensure that the elbows are soft and not hyperextended. When lying on the mat, be careful to take the ball only slightly overhead so as not to arch the back or lift the shoulders. Keep the knees bent if you have low-back pain and avoid the full roll-up, movement 2. If your back is fine and you're feeling quite strong, straighten the legs and flex the feet, pushing the heels away from the hips to add a hamstring stretch.

Purpose To strengthen the abdominals and learn to keep these muscles flat. To experience a hamstring stretch in movement 2.

Watchpoints • Be sure that the shoulder blades slide down the back. • Sink the navel into the spine as you roll up and down. • Do not arch the back when you take the ball overhead. If you suffer from a disc injury in the low back, avoid the full-flexion movement (movement 2).

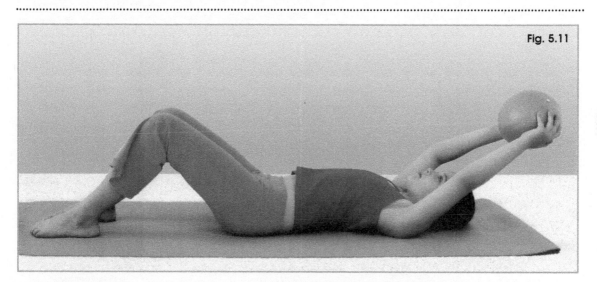

Fig. 5.11

starting position

Lie on your back, feet on the floor and legs together or slightly apart. Hold the ball between your hands. Keep the elbows soft. Keeping your shoulder blades on the mat, take the ball slightly overhead **(fig. 5.11)**.

movement 1: half roll-up

1. Inhale to lift the ball to the ceiling, head still on the mat **(fig. 5.12)**.
2. Exhale to sink the navel in and flex the body up, bringing the ball just above the knees. Keep the pelvis in neutral and the elbows soft **(fig. 5.13)**.

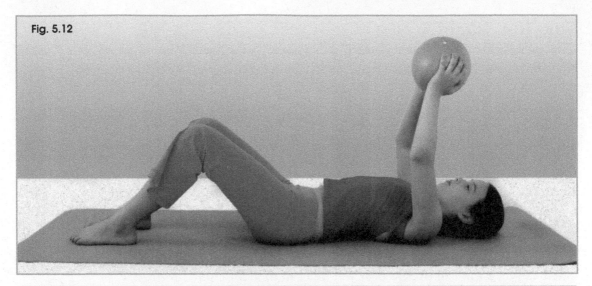

Fig. 5.12

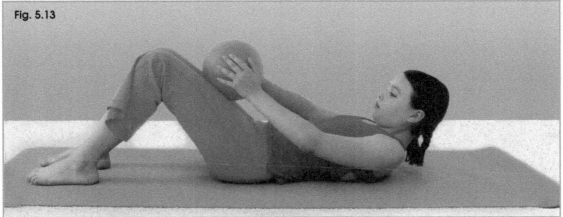

Fig. 5.13

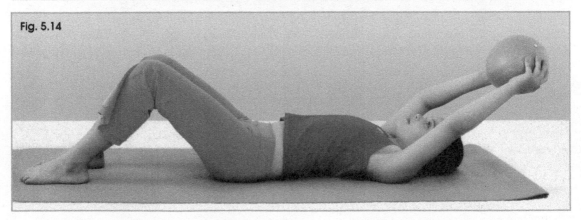

Fig. 5.14

3. Inhale to lift the arms back, but don't take them so far back that they go behind the ears. The gaze remains on your knees.

4. Exhale to roll back to the mat, arms returning slightly overhead **(fig. 5.14)**.

5. Repeat six to eight times.

movement 2: full roll-up (intermediate)

1. Stretch your legs long. Begin by holding the ball with the arms stretched slightly overhead. Inhale to lift the ball to the ceiling **(fig. 5.15)**.

2. Exhale to curl the body, peeling away from the mat one vertebra at a time **(fig. 5.16)**.

3. Inhale to extend the ball toward your toes **(fig. 5.17)** and start to roll back by pulling your navel toward your spine.

4. Exhale as you reverse the movement, rolling down one vertebra at a time.

5. When the shoulder blades return to the mat, the ball floats slightly back. Take care not to arch the back.

6. Repeat six to eight times.

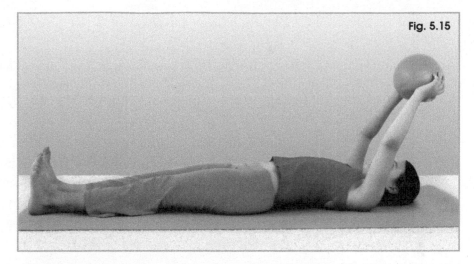

Fig. 5.15

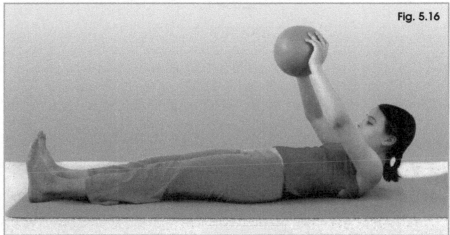

Fig. 5.16

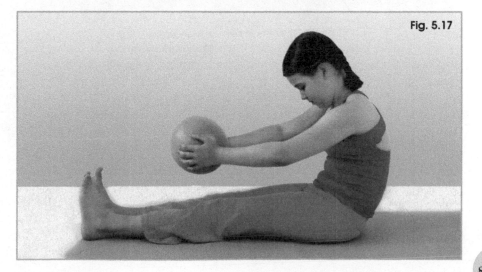

Fig. 5.17

Single- and Double-Leg Stretches

For the leg stretches the pelvis should move out of neutral and into a position in which the low back "imprints" or flattens down on the mat. Do not force the low back down: it will probably flatten naturally as the deep and superficial abdominals work together. What we do not want is overarching of the low back in these more challenging moves, so a slight "imprint" position is preferred when both legs come up in the air. If you have neck tension, do not use the ball and leave the head down on the mat. If you have low-back pain, keep the legs high in the air as you extend them. Small or large balls add upper body and abdominal challenge to these classic Pilates exercises. On the exhalation, squeeze the ball by pressing the palms of the hands against the side of the ball, putting equal pressure on both sides.

Purpose To work coordination, breathing, and abdominal strength.

Watchpoints • Keep ankles, hips, and knees in alignment. • Keep legs fully stretched, toes long but not tense. • The upper torso is stable; do not pull the shoulders from side to side or allow them to hunch up to your ears. • When your head is up, your gaze is on your knees, not on the ceiling.

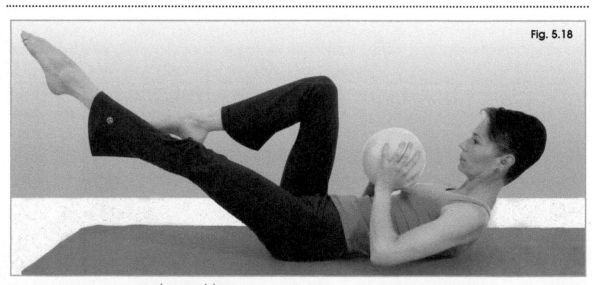

Fig. 5.18

starting position

Lie flat on your back, knees to chest. Hold a small ball on your knees.

movement 1: single-leg stretch

1. On the exhalation, curl the upper body upward as you simultaneously extend one leg 45 degrees from the floor. Squeeze the small ball and keep the elbows soft **(fig. 5.18)**.

2. Inhale to switch the legs slowly. Exhale to extend the second leg, squeezing the ball.

3. Repeat for five sets, or ten times with each leg. Then lower the head to the mat and pull the knees into the chest, resting the ball on the shins.

movement 2: double-leg stretch

1. If desired, switch to a large ball. Holding the ball on your knees, inhale to lift the head and bring the knees to the chest **(fig. 5.19)**.

2. Exhale to draw the navel inward and extend the legs and arms, arms in front of the ears or in line with them and legs 45 degrees or higher from the mat **(fig. 5.20)**.

3. Inhale to fold back in, bringing the ball to your shins or ankles. Exhale to stretch the legs and arms.

4. Repeat six to eight times. When the head is up the gaze should be on your knees, not on the ceiling. To finish, lower the head to the mat and pull the knees into the chest, resting the ball on the shins.

movement 3: modification

1. If you have low-back pain, extend the legs higher than 45 degrees. If you have neck tension leave your head down on the mat **(fig. 5.21)**.

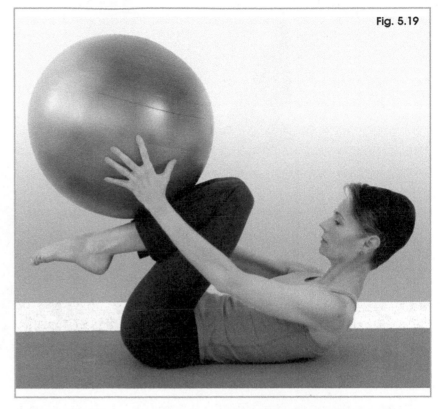

Fig. 5.19

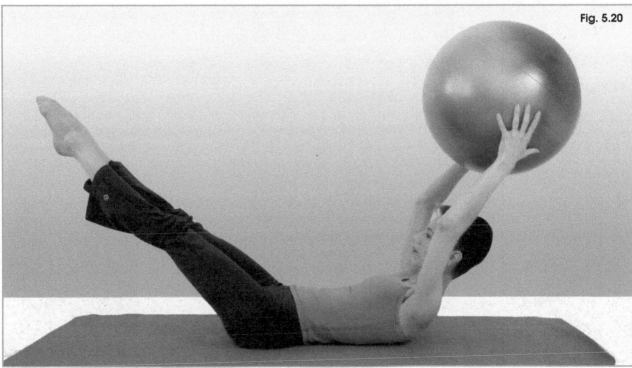

Fig. 5.20

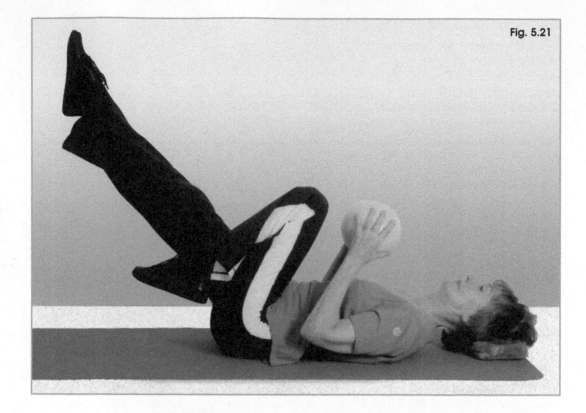

Fig. 5.21

Curling the Head off the Mat

When lifting the heavy head off the mat for abdominal work, keep three points in mind. First, make sure when lying on your back that your head is not tilted so far back that your neck overarches. Drop the chin gently forward, as if you want to hold a tennis ball at the throat. In some cases the head may need to rest on a flat pillow. Second, make sure the shoulders are down and not raised toward the ears. Finally, when you do lift the head, do so immediately, not as an afterthought. Some students may place hands lightly on the base of the skull to help guide the head, but use your abdominals—not your hands—to actually lift the head.

A resistance band or towel can be used to cradle the head and help people experience the proper way to lift the head. Lay the band or towel lengthwise on the center of the mat and lie back on it. Angle your elbows toward the ceiling and grab the band immediately above your head with your fingertips. On the exhalation, pull gently on the band; the head, cradled by the band or towel, will curl up. When the head is up your gaze should be on your knees, not on the ceiling.

Oblique Twists

The external and internal obliques, often referred to as the body's natural corset because of the way these muscles crisscross the torso, are responsible for sidebending and twisting of the spine. The obliques are traditionally weaker than the other abdominals. In this movement series try not to sidebend the torso; instead, pin one elbow back and slide the rib cage in the direction of the opposite hipbone. Resist the temptation to pull on the neck; in fact, keep the head heavy in the hands, elbows wide. Maintain the pelvis in neutral, though the low back may imprint down when you lift the legs in the air for the more challenging movement 2. Again, as in Single- and Double-Leg Stretches, the low back flattens to the mat to prevent it from overarching when the legs come up in the air. It is crucial that the pelvis does not rock from side to side. To test this, squeeze the legs together and place them in the air in the tabletop position for movement 2. Then place the small ball on the shins and balance the ball!

Purpose To tone the oblique muscles.

Watchpoints • Hands are placed lightly at the base of the skull; elbows reach to the side. • Keep the tailbone down on the mat and try not to rock the pelvis. • Keep the abs flat.

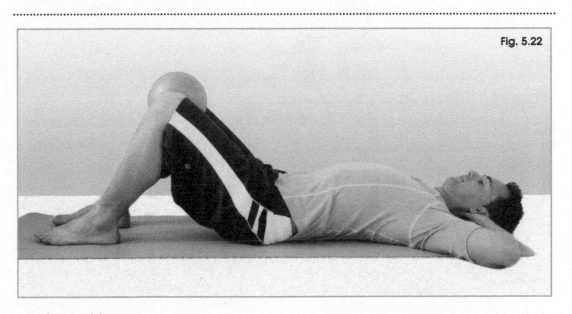

Fig. 5.22

starting position

Lie on your back with the ball positioned between your knees. Feet remain flat on the mat. Hands are behind the ears, elbows wide **(fig. 5.22)**.

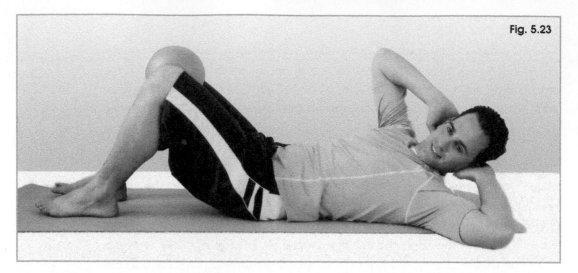

Fig. 5.23

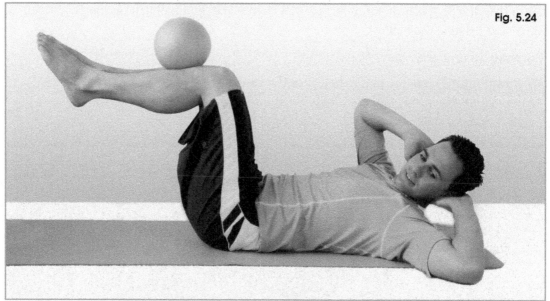

Fig. 5.24

movement 1: feet on the mat

1. Keeping your pelvis in neutral, on the exhalation pin your left elbow to the mat and slide your right rib cage toward the opposite hipbone. Gently squeeze the small ball **(fig. 5.23)**.

2. Inhale to return the head to the mat.

3. Repeat eight to ten times on each side.

movement 2: tabletop legs

1. Place your legs in tabletop position, knees and ankles together and small ball on your shins. Your low back will imprint on the mat.

2. On the exhalation pin your left elbow back and slide your right rib cage toward the opposite hipbone. Keep the small ball steady **(fig. 5.24)**.

3. Inhale to stay.

4. Exhale to return the head to the mat.

5. Repeat eight to ten times on each side.

With the Small Ball

Adapted from the small Pilates Barrel, movements 1 and 2 are fun *and* effective abdominal exercises. Imagine that you are moving the limbs through wet cement as you create a strong center against the movement of the heavy legs. The small ball should rest comfortably under the pelvis and not in the low back; a small portion of the ball may bulge out from under your tailbone when you are in the correct position. If desired, a percussive breath can be added to movement 2 as you inhale for three short "sniffs" and exhale for three short "blows." For movements 3 and 4, your hips should be stacked one on top of another.

Purpose To strengthen the abdominals. To tone the legs and buttocks.

Watchpoints • Hold the navel-to-spine connection to keep the low back imprinted on the ball. • To make movement 1, bicycle, more difficult, keep the knees farther away from the core of the body; to make it easier, bring the knees in closer to the abs. In movements 3 and 4, don't take the legs high. • You should not feel pain in your waist.

starting position

Lie on the mat with your feet on the mat. Lift the pelvis and tuck the small ball under your pelvis. Bring your bent knees up toward your chest. Let your weight sink into the ball. Your neck should be relaxed; you should feel no pressure on it.

movement 1: bicycle in air

1. Straighten your legs into the air, toes long. Gently draw the navel in toward the spine **(fig. 5.25)**.
2. Breathing naturally, draw

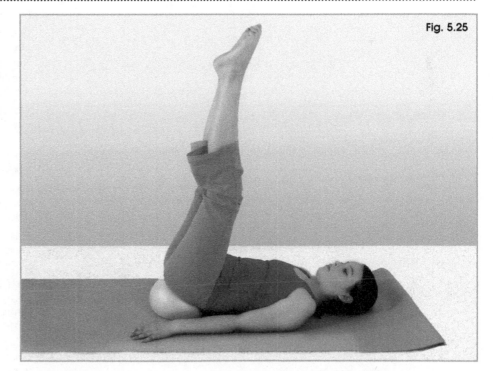

Fig. 5.25

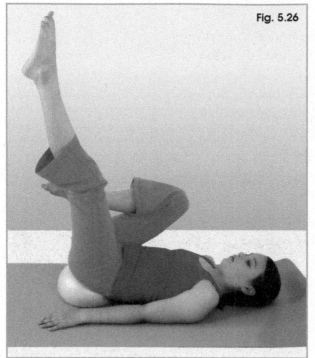

Fig. 5.26

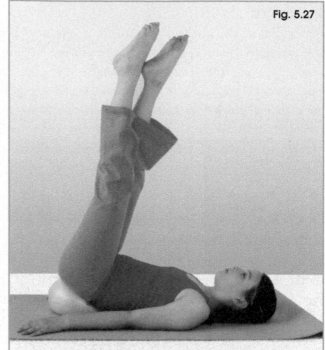

Fig. 5.27

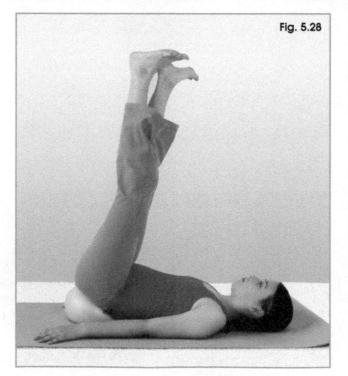

Fig. 5.28

one leg down to begin moving your legs in a bicycling motion. Turn the bicycle wheel smoothly five times in one direction **(fig. 5.26)**.
3. Reverse the rotation of the wheel for five spins. Breathe naturally.

movement 2: beats

1. Straighten your legs into the air, toes long. Turning both legs out from the hip sockets, cross the right leg onto the front of the left thigh. Gently draw the navel inward **(fig. 5.27)**.
2. On three short inhalations, cross the right leg in front of the left thigh and back and forth three times.
3. Flex the feet. On three short exhales, cross the legs three times back and forth **(fig. 5.28)**.
4. Repeat for six sets.

movement 3: on the side, squeeze and lift

1. Lie on your side and place the ball between your ankles. Make a long line from the head through the shoulders, hips, and feet. Your head can be propped up by your hand or relaxed on the mat. If possible, lift your upper body up and out of the waist **(fig. 5.29)**.
2. On the exhalation squeeze the small ball and lift both legs a couple of inches from the mat **(fig. 5.30)**.
3. Inhale to lower. Exhale to lift. Repeat eight times. Turn over and do the same movement on the other side.

movement 4: on the side, inner thighs

1. To isolate the inner thigh of the bottom leg, bring the top leg across the body and prop a small ball under the top leg to ensure alignment of the pelvis. Then completely relax the top leg and focus on the inner thigh of the bottom leg.
2. On the exhalation, pulse the bottom leg, keeping the leg straight **(fig. 5.31)**.
3. Then, using the same leg, make six to eight circles in one direction. Then reverse.
4. Repeat the movement on the other side.

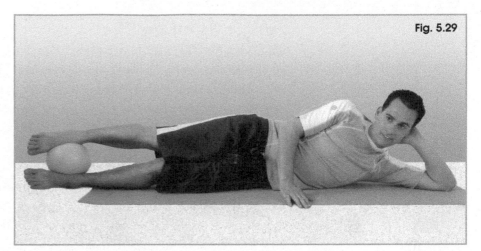

Fig. 5.29

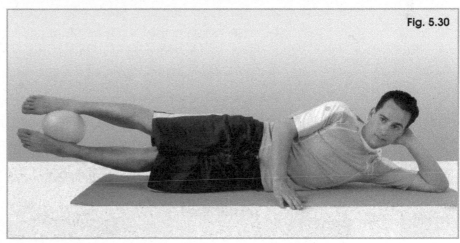

Fig. 5.30

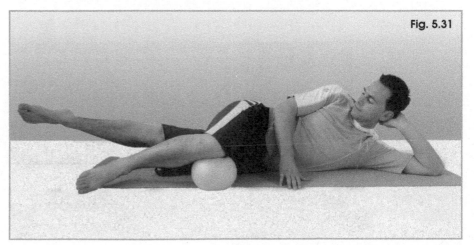

Fig. 5.31

Ab Curls on the Ball

Dr. Stuart McGill, a leading expert on low-back disorders, found that a curl-up performed on a ball with the feet on the ground virtually doubled the abdominal-muscle activation of a curl-up performed on a stable surface. In working with these exercises, notice how the abdominals contract and then lengthen as you perform your repetitions, remembering that the eccentric contraction (lengthening back onto the ball) is more work for the muscles. Movement 2 focuses on the isometric contraction, designed for building endurance. Breathing naturally, maintain the body in its curled-up position, increasing the tension in the muscle without changing its length. To make the exercise less difficult, walk your feet a few steps in front of the ball, dropping the buttocks slightly. To make it more difficult, narrow the base of support so that the feet are close together. Even coming out of this exercise—moving the body from a horizontal to seated position—is in itself a fantastic abdominal exercise. But this maneuver may be challenging for a beginner. Have a friend spot you the first time—see the box on page 214.

Purpose To strengthen the upper and the superficial abdominals.

Watchpoints • If possible, keep the buttocks lifted to the same height as the thighs and knees. • Do not pull on your neck or dig your chin into your chest when you curl up.

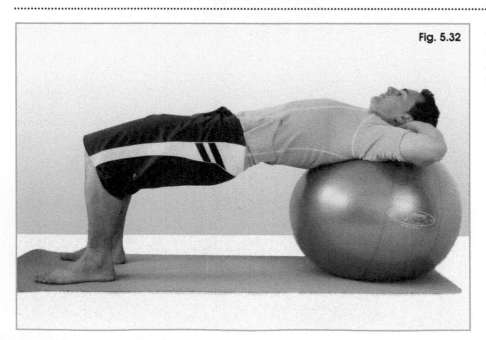

Fig. 5.32

starting position

Sit on the center of your ball. Slowly walk your feet away from the ball; the ball will roll under you. Walk the feet out until the shoulders are resting comfortably on the ball. Place the hands behind the ears **(fig. 5.32)**.

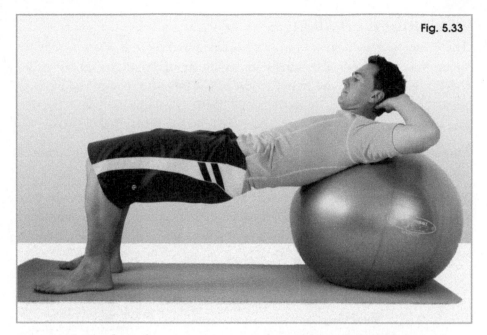

Fig. 5.33

movement 1: ab curls

1. Inhale to prepare, keeping the elbows reaching out to the sides.
2. Exhale to pull your navel inward and curl the upper body. The lower back is off the ball **(fig. 5.33)**.
3. Inhale and stay. Exhale to lower the upper body to the ball.
4. Inhale to lengthen back, feeling the abdominals stretch.
5. Repeat eight times.

movement 2: with hold

1. Inhale to prepare, keeping the elbows reaching out to the sides.
2. Exhale to pull your navel inward and curl the upper body. The lower back is off the ball.
3. Inhale, exhale, and inhale, holding for a few counts.
4. Exhale to lower the upper body to the ball. Lengthen back and feel the abdominals stretch.
5. Repeat eight times.
6. To come out of position, put your hands behind your head and lift the head, bringing the chin to the chest. Walk your feet slowly toward the ball. Place your hands on the top of the ball to aid you as you sit up on the ball. This may not be easy for some beginners. You may have to lower your buttocks to the ground instead to come out of this exercise.

Abdominal Challenges

These exercises are a great finish to the abdominal series if you are ready for them. Make sure your abdominals are strong enough that you do not strain the low back and be sure that you are well warmed up before you attempt these challenging moves. In movement 2, think of peeling away from the mat one vertebra at a time, using the abdominals and not the arms.

Purpose Movement 1 strengthens the abdominal obliques. Movement 2 strengthens the upper and lower abdominals.

Watchpoints • Keep your movements smooth, using the abdominals—not momentum. • Maintain the navel-to-spine connection. • Keep your head aligned on the spine and do not look from side to side. • Do not put too much weight on the neck in movement 2.

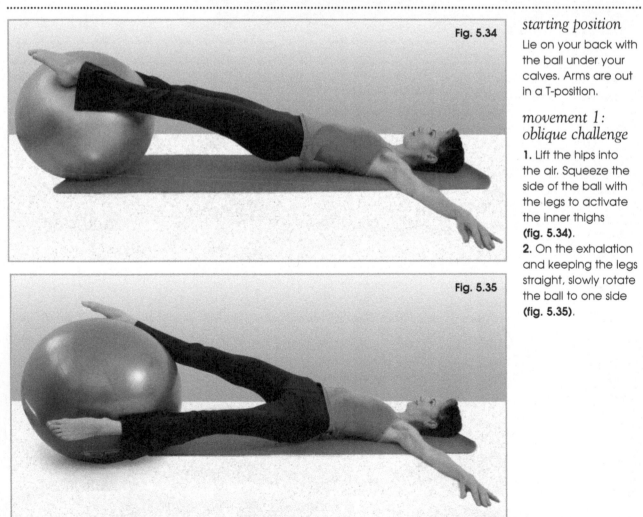

Fig. 5.34

Fig. 5.35

starting position

Lie on your back with the ball under your calves. Arms are out in a T-position.

movement 1: oblique challenge

1. Lift the hips into the air. Squeeze the side of the ball with the legs to activate the inner thighs **(fig. 5.34)**.
2. On the exhalation and keeping the legs straight, slowly rotate the ball to one side **(fig. 5.35)**.

3. Bring the ball back to center and then roll to the opposite side.

4. Repeat six times each side. For extra challenge, lift the arms straight up in the air.

movement 2: abdominal challenge (intermediate)

1. Pick up the ball between the feet, lift it in the air, and take it into the hands. Place the ball behind your head. Keeping your hands on the side of the ball, lower the legs as low as you can while keeping the low back on the mat **(fig. 5.36)**.

2. On the exhalation squeeze the abdominals and slowly take the legs overhead. If possible, touch the ball with your toes **(fig. 5.37)**.

3. Inhale to take the toes an inch or two deeper over the ball. Exhale to return the legs to the start position; move the ball to an angle at which you are able to keep your lower back on the mat **(fig. 5.38)**.

4. Repeat six times.

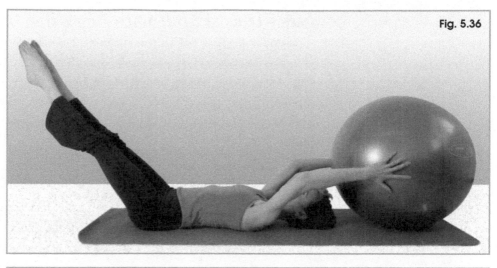

Fig. 5.36

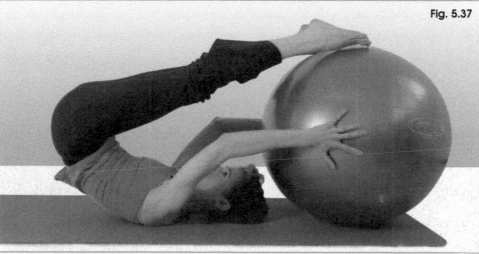

Fig. 5.37

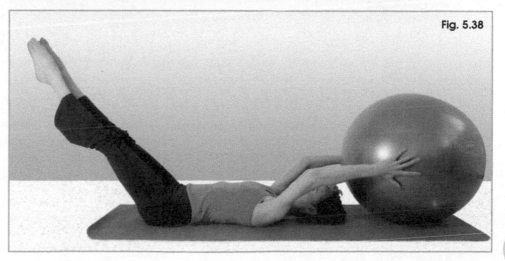

Fig. 5.38

101

Side-Twist Plank with Leg Lift

The entire body works in this ultimate core challenge. From a strong plank position you will swivel your body as a unit and line up your hipbones one on top of the other, perpendicular to the floor. When your body feels "stiff as a board," lift the top leg to add an extra challenge to the oblique muscle. Ensure your navel-to-spine connection to keep the middle of the body from sagging and to keep the low back safe.

Purpose To work the abdominals, the upper body, and the abdominal obliques.

Watchpoints • Maintain good stability in the shoulder girdle. • Keep your shoulder blades open across the back and down, not up by your ears. • Keep your gaze down on the mat. • Keep both arms straight when you swivel the torso.

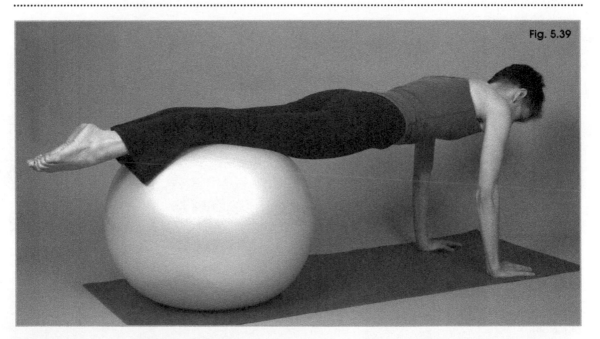

Fig. 5.39

starting position

Kneel in front of the ball. Place hands palm down on the mat and walk out until the ball is on the thighs or, for extra challenge, the shins. Fingertips should be parallel to the body, elbows angled slightly back. Keep the legs very straight with the buttocks working and the navel lifted **(fig. 5.39)**.

movement 1: side-twist plank (intermediate)

1. Keeping your head and shoulders exactly where they are, swivel the lower body until you lift one hip and place it directly on top of the other. Legs and arms are straight. Your gaze is on the mat **(fig. 5.40)**.
2. Hold for a few seconds, breathing naturally.

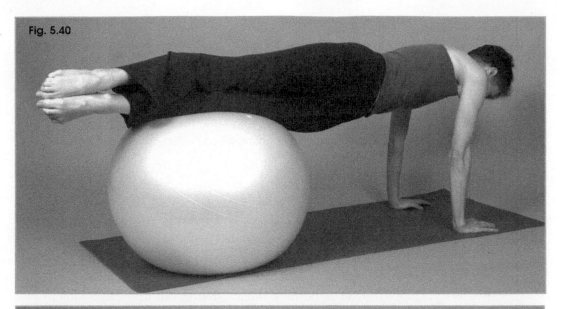

Fig. 5.40

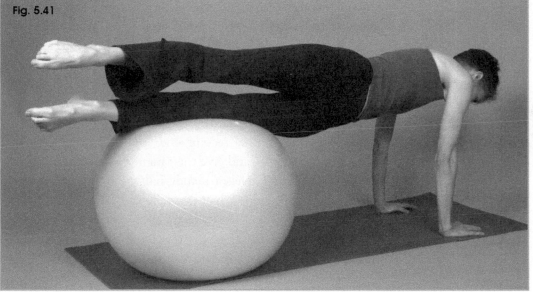

Fig. 5.41

3. Return to plank position and swivel to the other side.

4. Repeat two or three times each side. Then pick the hands up and walk them back to the ball and rest over the ball.

movement 2: side-twist plank with leg lift (intermediate)

1. Begin by setting up the body exactly as in movement 1.

2. After you have lined up one hip on top of the other, lift the top leg two inches. Hold for two or three counts, breathing naturally **(fig. 5.41)**.

3. Return to plank position and swivel to the other side, then lift the top leg.

4. Repeat two or three times each side. Then pick the hands up and walk them back to the ball and rest over the ball.

In the next chapter we will start on an effective and safe weight-training program to help you stay youthful and strong. The heavy leather belt used by bodybuilders is not necessary. Instead, you will use your own deep inner belt—the musculature of the powerhouse—to support the midsection when you lift.

The abdomen is particularly vulnerable to aging. Gravity and overeating take their tolls. The check-in below will help those of you who are watching what you eat preserve muscle and bone as you strengthen your body.

Check In: Dieting Blues

All the abdominal exercises in the world will not help you lose weight if you do not adjust your diet. Adjusting your diet does not necessarily mean cutting back, as many researchers are finding that cutting calories too drastically can trigger hormonal shifts that make the body believe it is starving and will conserve calories instead of burning them. Dieting can also cause muscle loss. *Strong Women Stay Slim* authors Miriam Nelson, Ph.D., and Sarah Wernick, Ph.D., claim that when women diet at least 25 to 30 percent of the weight they shed isn't fat at all, but water, muscle, bone, and lean tissue. To move the body we need energy, and energy comes from the food we eat. But if you eat more than you can burn off, fat accumulates. Not overnight either. It is not one good dinner out a week that puts on weight but an imbalance between how much you consume and how much you burn.

Strong Women Stay Slim authors recommend strength training to help women preserve and tone muscles and give their metabolic rate a boost while they lose weight. In Dr. Miriam E. Nelson's study, half the women did strength training twice a week while the other half just followed individualized diets. Nelson found that the diet-only volunteers lost an average of thirteen pounds during her study. The women who strength trained lost about the same amount. What is significant is the body composition. The women in the diet-only group lost lean tissue—mainly muscle—along with fat. The women who did strength training actually gained pounds of lean tissue (1.4 pounds) and lost 44 percent more fat than the diet-only group.

Because women are already vulnerable to bone loss and they have a tendency to lose lean tissue and muscles along with fat, strict dieting is not the solution. Instead eat food rich in protein and fiber and combine proper-sized meals with exercise and strength training. Many sports nutritionists recommend 40 percent carbohydrates, 30 percent protein, and 30 percent fat in each meal. Carbohydrates, especially fruits and vegetables, energize the body. Watch out for the other carbs—potatoes, pastas, and breads—which make you tired. Proteins are the building blocks of the body: poultry, lean meats, and fish fall into this category. If your body can tolerate dairy, nonfat milk and yogurt are good dietary sources of calcium and vitamin D. Then there are the so-called good fats, the sources of which come from animals and plants. These fats are essential to the body—they assist in energy production and improve skin quality. These fats are found in avocados, nuts, flax seed, grapeseed, good olive oils, and oily fish. Bad fats, which are often used in processed foods, clog the arteries and contribute to endless health problems.

What is needed is a realistic plan for eating well coupled with exercise that you enjoy and can do safely. Keep nutritious and filling foods on hand (especially fiber-rich fruits, vegetables, legumes, and whole grains) and cut back on sweets, bad fats, and salt. Always eat a small portion and chew and drink slowly: the digestive system can be dramatically improved by drinking two liters of water a day and chewing your food properly. Make sure you are eating enough—you need food for energy and to alleviate depression and lethargy. A substantial breakfast and a satisfying lunch is highly recommended so that you don't spiral into binge eating. Buy a lunchbox or small cooler and carry nourishing snacks around with you at all times. Experiment with new cuisines to aid you in eating at least five portions of fresh fruit and three portions of vegetables a day.

Throw out your diet books and start eating like a human being. Read something inspiring like Dr. Andrew Weil's *Eating Well for Optimum Health: The Essential Guide to Bringing Health and Pleasure Back to Eating* (Quill, 2001) or Victoria Moran's *Fit from Within* (Contemporary Books, 2002).

6
Strength Training and Antiaging

The Long Slow Goodbye of Aging

I recall the exact moment. I was four months shy of my fortieth birthday, playing outside with my oldest niece, and I could not pull myself up on the monkey bars. I stopped almost before I began. I was winded and had strained something in the back of my buttocks. What was I thinking? For two decades I hadn't done anything really physical except take long walks. Now my body was too tight to lift my legs up to the platform. I could not scoot under the bar. Nor did I have the upper-body strength to heave myself up from one level to the next. My inabilities shocked me.

Almost a decade later I am at a lake with my younger niece. I sprawl on my belly, roll, slither, and snake my way through alligator and other shallow-water games. I haul great piles of sand for sand castles, crawling on my hands and knees for hours. I am nearly ten years older than I was at the time of that wake-up call on the monkey bars, yet physically I feel many years younger. I am almost fifty now, yet I can easily slide a hefty carry-on into an airplane's overhead bin; I can build a ten-pail sand castle and squat back on my heels to enjoy it. For me this is what true fitness means—it's not about having chiseled muscles or about how much you can bench-press. Functional movement and strength are the gifts of my Pilates career—begun when I was forty but poised to benefit me for many years to come.

As we age, maintaining function and strength are paramount to preserving quality of life. An inactive lifestyle is hazardous to your health and, by example, the health of those close to you. The road of least resistance leads to what yoga author Stephen Cope dubs the "long slow goodbye of aging."

There are many advantages to aging. We mellow with age, accepting ourselves and others with greater grace and compassion. Our minds know more, confidence is greater, and there is real potential for career growth. Retirement is thought of as a time of freedom but, ironically, many people are not at all free in their "golden years." Their minds and their financial health may be sound, but sadly their bodies are in a great state of decline. How could this have happened?

The aging process affects us differently in our thirties, forties, fifties, sixties, and later, and there is also a significant difference in the ways men age and the ways women age. In their earlier years men are plagued by sports-related or sometimes war-related injuries and risk-taking behavior. In their middle years, the stress and responsibilities of family and career take their toil. In their later years, decline in testosterone levels and inactivity lead to a decline in vitality and strength. Major causes of death for men after age sixty-five are lung cancer, heart disease, stroke, and prostate cancer.

Women live longer than men and their aging process is different because of hormonal fluctuations. A woman's twenties and thirties may be focused around childbearing and postpartum experiences that can make women vulnerable to weight gain and extra stress. Raising children while juggling jobs and other obligations takes its toll. In the forties, perimenopause begins and with it comes heavy menstruation, fluctuating estrogen levels, and (often) weight gain. In addition, women lose about one-third of a pound of muscle each year.

Into her fifties a woman's metabolism continues to slow, and she has to work harder not to let body fat take the place of lost muscle. Menopause signals the end of reproductive life and decreased levels of estrogen in the body. Bone health and skeletal disease become a considerable concern. Osteoporosis, fragility, fractures, and collapsed vertebrae can go hand in hand.

Despite these differences in the aging process, both men and women do share this reality: all age-associated declines are not inevitable. Much research supports strength training as having a significant impact on turning back the clock, even for adults in their seventies and eighties. If you are concerned about the manner in which you feel your body aging, you have to ask yourself this: "Should I continue on the road of least resistance, or should I make the changes necessary to postpone or delay the effects of aging?"

stress, depression, heart health, and weight training

There are benefits to weight training other than just seeing your muscles develop and feeling them growing stronger.

Exercise increases serotonin levels, releases adrenalin, and boosts energy and endurance. It is known to help sleep patterns and to boost your immune system. It is an excellent stress buster.

Dr. Richard Friedman, a doctor interviewed by Gina Kolata for her book *Ultimate Fitness*, spoke about the effects of strength training on depression. Lift weights, he advised his patients, calling the actual effort of weight lifting a "pleasure."

Research has shown that weight lifting can also improve cardiovascular function for men and women. According to an American Heart Association survey, weight training two or three times a week can improve glucose metabolism and can reduce blood pressure and the chance of developing diabetes. Strength training was found to be beneficial to some patients who had had heart attacks.

*Age has never harmed
anyone, nor has it ever
killed a single human being.
It is what happens during the
aging process that harms and
kills human beings.*
—Thomas Hanna

The Antiaging Benefits of Strength Training

Why would someone find the lifting of hand weights or machine resistance anything but a toiling chore? You need to try it to understand. There is a pleasure and an intensity to lifting weights: your muscles immediately feel warm and alive. You start by thinking, "I'm not in the mood to lift weights." But then you begin and something clicks in, eventually clearing your head and leaving your body with an intense feeling of release. Even pulling a resistance band feels like a shot to the heart. The muscles fatigue, relax, and warm up. After a series of repetitions you experience a burst of energy; after a full session you sleep better at night.

The most important gift of strength training is that it directly affects your functional movement. It is not just a pleasure enhancer and a stress buster. The result is strength you can use immediately to carry children or grandchildren, climb stairs, and keep up on walks.

Researchers at Tufts University have shown that men and women in their sixties who lifted weights strengthened their muscles by 100 to 175 percent. Dr. Walter Frontera had his volunteers work at 80 percent of their capacity; in just twelve weeks the muscles that were exercised became 10 to 12 percent larger. Another group of Tufts scientists had remarkable results in a nursing-home group of frail participants who ranged from ages eighty-six to ninety-six: in eight weeks they increased their strength by 175 percent. Some residents discarded their canes, and walking speed and balance rose by an average of 48 percent.

Dr. Miriam E. Nelson, in whose book *Strong Women Stay Young* these findings are published, expanded this research and worked with a younger group of women. Nelson recruited forty healthy but sedentary postmenopausal women. Half the women maintained their usual lifestyle; the other half came to her lab twice a week and lifted weights. After strength training twice a week for a year, the bodies of the women in the second group were fifteen to twenty years more youthful. Bone loss was prevented or reversed and flexibility and balance improved. In addition, Dr. Nelson reported that the women "felt happier, more energetic, and more self-confident."

Some evidence suggests that people lose fast-twitch muscles as part of the aging process; other research suggests that fast-twitch muscle becomes slow-twitch as we age. Most researchers agree that all muscles of the body possess some of each type of muscle, but the ratio of fast-twitch to slow-twitch depends on the function required of the muscle. Regardless of age, strength training improves performance of the muscles and the ability of a given muscle to contract. And it does not take long to see a difference in your body. The women in Dr. Nelson's study who did not lift weights aged, whereas the women who lifted weights became more active and had better balance and flexibility.

Dr. Nelson also discovered that the weight-lifting women in her study ended up with less fat and more muscle. Even though this was not one of the objectives of the study, Dr. Nelson found that lifting weights boosts calorie-burning power. As people age, muscles shrink and fat accumulates. "Muscle is active tissue and consumes calories," notes Nelson. "Stored fat, on the other hand, is inert and uses very little energy."

For older adults, especially women, perhaps the most important benefit of weight training is bone health. As women move through menopause their bones change dramatically and silently. This creates a dangerous, yet preventable, situation.

Osteoporosis—The Silent Bone Saboteur

Following menopause, one in two women will experience an osteoporotic fracture during her remaining lifetime! This sobering fact was told by Dr. Ethel C. Siris in New York City at a seminar held by the Society for Women's Health Research. According to Dr. Siris, 25 percent will have a vertebral fracture and 15 percent will have a hip fracture. Osteoporosis affects mainly women over age fifty, but it also can affect men as well.

Osteoporosis is a preventable disease. In youth our bodies are programmed to accumulate bone. This is why good diet and exercise is so essential for teens and why resistance training benefits youth as much as older people. Remind your children, grandchildren, and the young people around you that their present diet and exercise habits will affect them much later in life. Encourage them to take up bone-stressing play like skipping and hopscotch or activities such as dancing or track and field and to try some of the exercises in this book.

You build bone up to age thirty and then you lose bone. The rate of loss is slow at first. After menopause, however, most women lose bone fast as calcium absorption and estrogen levels decline. This creates an imbalance between bone reabsorption and bone formation, a condition that leads to thin and porous bones. Women who have smaller bodies and bone mass to begin with are particularly vulnerable to osteoporosis. There is a higher incidence of osteoporosis in white and Asian women; in women who have had ovaries surgically removed or who experience early menopause; in women with a family history of osteoporosis; in thin women with small bones; in women who smoke; and in women with a history of no exercise or obsessive exercise to the point that their menstrual cycles were affected.

Hormone replacement therapy (HRT) has been shown to offer women bone protection; however, the latest controversy around the possible health risk of long-term HRT has challenged women to rethink this option. The Women's Health Initiative study ended early when it became clear that the risks of Prempro, a popular hormone replacement, overshadowed its benefits.

There are other options to combat osteoporosis, this silent and invisible saboteur. The first step is to take a bone-density test and have a plan of action that includes appropriate medical treatment, diet, and exercise. A bone-density test is a safe and painless way to measure the thickness of your bones and determine whether you have osteoporosis or osteopenia, the beginning states of this disease. If you are in menopause or have some of the risk factors mentioned above, ask your doctor to prescribe this fifteen-minute test. For some women the test provides a baseline; for others it generates the motivation to make a lifestyle or diet change. Recommended daily calcium intake for menopausal women who are trying to prevent osteoporosis is 1,200 to 1,500 milligrams a day, including 400 IUs of vitamin D a day to increase calcium absorption. Good dietary sources of calcium include hard cheese, low-fat and nonfat milk and yogurt, tofu, canned salmon with its bones, and calcium-fortified orange juice.

Strength training can prevent and reverse the effects of osteoporosis and alleviate some of the discomforts of menopause without the side effects of drugs. Aim for thirty minutes of strength training three times a week in addition to walking or other aerobic exercise. Dr. Nelson incrementally and progressively increased the amount of resistance in her test with postmenopausal women. She also advocates the benefits of high-impact exercise—jumping rope and vertical jumping—for women who have joints strong enough to withstand the impact.

Light Versus Heavy Weights

Joseph Pilates lived well into his eighties. In pictures of him in his last years we see a lean and fit man—a testimony to the antiaging benefits of his exercises. Joseph Pilates used various springs and pulleys to add resistance to his work, not to isolate and overload a muscle into exhaustion but to build long and lean muscles—as opposed to bulk—and to train the body functionally with light weights.

A Pilates approach to strength training keeps the muscles in balance. Low levels of resistance minimize strain on joints and soft tissues and are better for those returning to exercise or recovering from injuries. In traditional weight training the emphasis is on how much weight can be lifted; often this translates to moving a heavy weight in one fixed direction. In the Pilates Method lighter weights are used but you consciously add resistance to the weights, meaning you engage your muscles, pressing the weights smoothly and often slowly as if moving the limbs through wet cement. With this approach you have the choice to move the weights slower or faster, change direction, and move the arms through different planes.

Most important of all in Strength Training on the Ball is the fact that we are not just lifting weights but are also using weights in conjunction with the instability of the ball. When working on a mobile surface, the use of gravity and body weight adds additional challenge to the exercise. Moreover, lighter weights give freedom to work in the full range of motion—to rotate the arms inward or outward, to make circles or diagonals, and to otherwise work the body as a unit. An integrated approach creates a much more balanced body.

You may, however, decide to lift heavier weights. When using heavier weights, extreme care must be taken with alignment and technique and to give yourself time to adapt to increased loads. Soreness can develop after a strenuous weight-lifting session. Sometimes this comes in the form of a delayed muscle tenderness that develops twelve to twenty-four hours after the workout. To prevent soreness, progress gradually, making sure you warm up adequately and stretch gently after lifting. Give yourself adequate rest periods after using heavier weights. Make the day after lifting a day of rest—during this recovery period energy is replenished and lactic acid is removed from the muscles. Moderate exercise such as walking and stretching on the day of rest is more beneficial than total inactivity.

The Pilates-Based Arm Work

As you begin weight training, be on the lookout for signs of muscle fatigue. There should be no uncomfortable sensations within the muscle such as cramping or pain. Make sure you are able to complete your reps in good alignment and with a smooth quality of movement. Jerky motions or substituting the work of one muscle for another must be avoided.

The small muscles that run from the spine to the shoulder blades are extremely important in "fixing" or stabilizing the blades. So are the muscles that link the arm to the shoulder to ensure correct arm position. These exercises target the stabilizers to prevent injuries or other problems in the future, as well as work the more superficial muscles of the arm and shoulder.

To use a ball as a bench, you need good balance. For that reason, the following exercises may not be for everyone. Practice the balance tests in the check-in at the end of chapter 4 and perform the following exercises first in

The Three Types of Muscle Contraction

*W*hen you lift a weight there is more going on than simply muscle pulling bone. The nervous system gathers information and sends an electrochemical impulse from the brain down your spinal column, signaling the muscle fibers to contract. The skeletal muscles are made up of bundles of muscles fibers, which are in turn made up of extremely long, thin myofibrils. When the muscles are stimulated by a nerve signal, a series of chemical reactions take place in the muscle, causing the muscle to fire. Imagine putting one hand over another on a thick rope and sliding something toward you. This is how a muscle "fires," or contracts.

There are three types of muscular contractions. In the example of the arm curl, the bicep contracts into a shortened position when you bring a weight up to your shoulder. This is called a *concentric contraction*. The second contraction is the *eccentric action*, when the muscles lengthen under load in a controlled way, as the bicep does when returning the weight back down to your side. Finally, there is the *isometric contraction*, where you increase the tension in the muscle without changing its length. An example would be holding the leg up, a foot or two from the ground, without movement. In this position the thigh muscles work hard against the resistance of your body's weight. Pushing or pulling a stationary object can also be an isometric exercise. The isometric contraction builds endurance in the muscle as well as improves strength.

Varying the amount of time the muscle spends in each type of contraction can influence strength gains. The careful use of these three different actions is important in a Pilates approach.

the position shown in movement 9, the modification. A Physio Roll will give you more support than a ball because it rolls only in one direction.

Ball as Bench

Because you are working on a mobile surface and moving the arms through a full range of motion, you will not be able to load up with heavy weights. Begin with 1- or 2-pound weights. Later you can increase to 3- or 5-pound weights if desired. Lying back on the ball will set you up for a fuller movement range, more than you could get on a mat and more comfortably than on a bench. Your head, neck, and shoulders are totally supported on the ball, but the low back is off the ball to work the buttocks. Keep the hips lifted and remember to engage the abdominal powerhouse before you lift by drawing the navel in toward the spine to protect the low back. The center of the kneecap should track over the second toe; the feet are parallel and hip-distance apart. If your back begins to hurt, drop your tailbone down into the squat position and perform the arm work here. This modification (see page 123) puts the body in good alignment and takes strain off the low back. To add significant challenge to these exercises, perform them with eyes closed or with one foot on a small ball or another unstable surface, such as a wobble board.

Purpose Movements 1 and 2, the chest press, work the pectorals and triceps; the single-arm work requires the obliques and deep rotators of the spine to stabilize the rib cage. Movements 3 and 4 work the deltoids and pectorals. Movement 5, triceps isolator, works the triceps muscles of your upper arms; movement 6 works the biceps. Movements 7 and 8 work the pectorals, intercostals, serratus, and abdominals.

Watchpoints • Make sure your head and neck are totally supported by the ball, not hanging backward. • For chest press and flies, keep your weights at heart level; don't let them drift up to head level. • When extending the arms, don't lock the elbows: keep the elbows slightly bent in the top position. • Keep the abdominals tight and the buttock muscles activated to keep the hips working against gravity. • Keep the shoulder blades in place. • Use only one 2-, 3-, or 5-pound weight for movements 7 and 8. • If your low back begins to hurt, use the modification shown in movement 9.

starting position

Sit on your ball. Walk your feet out and let the ball roll under you until your head and neck are totally supported by the ball. Hips are up; abdominals are engaged.

movement 1: chest press

1. Start with weights resting on the side of your chest, just above the armpits. The palms face forward **(fig. 6.1)**. Inhale to prepare.

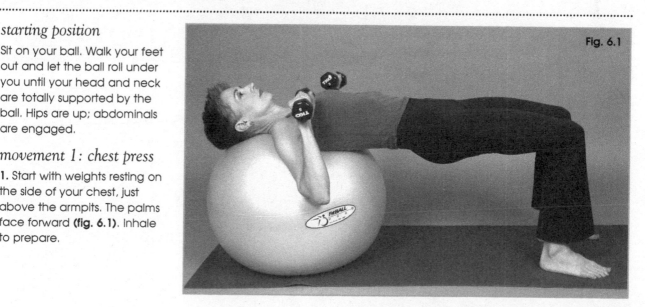

Fig. 6.1

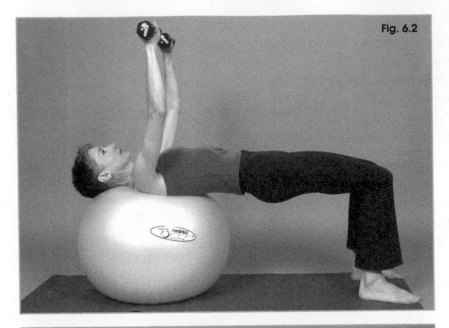

Fig. 6.2

2. Exhale to raise the arms up to shoulder level, keeping the shoulder blades on the ball **(fig. 6.2)**.
3. Repeat eight to ten times. Then try the same exercise with palms facing inward.

movement 2: single-arm chest press

1. Place the weight in your left hand. Start with the left hand resting on the side of your chest just above the armpit. The palms face forward. Place your right hand on your forehead **(fig. 6.3)** or raise your right arm directly above your shoulder as a counterbalance.
2. On the exhalation raise your left arm, keeping your body steady on the ball **(fig. 6.4)**.

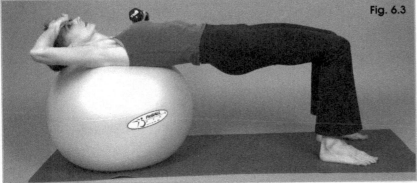

Fig. 6.3

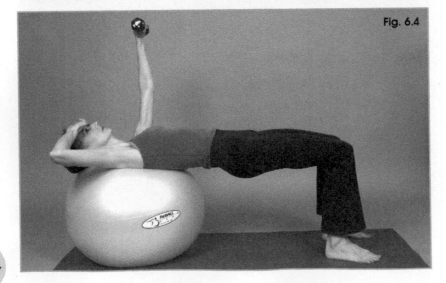

Fig. 6.4

3. Repeat eight to ten times. Then perform the same exercise with the other arm.

4. For a challenging variation, bend the knees to squat and place one foot on a small ball **(fig. 6.5)**. Roll back onto the ball, ensuring that the neck and head are totally supported. Place your left hand on your forehead or raise it directly above your shoulder as a counterbalance **(fig. 6.6)**, then exhale and raise your right arm **(fig. 6.7)**. Repeat eight to ten times.

5. Come out, move the small ball to the opposite foot, and set yourself up for the second side.

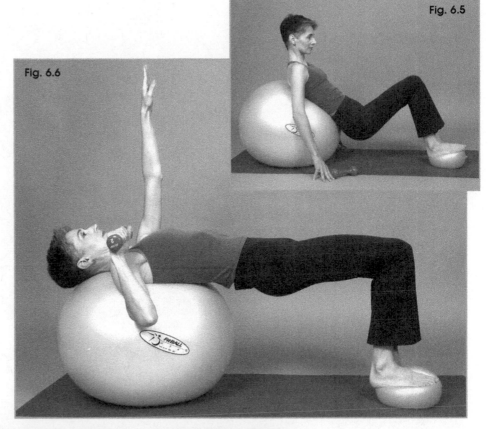

Fig. 6.5

Fig. 6.6

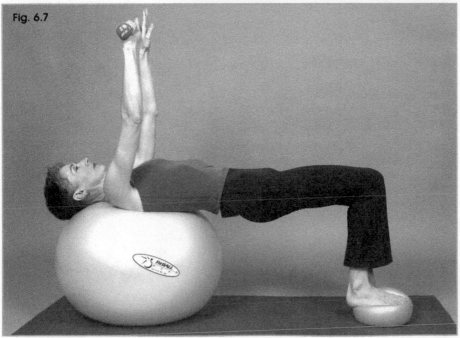

Fig. 6.7

115

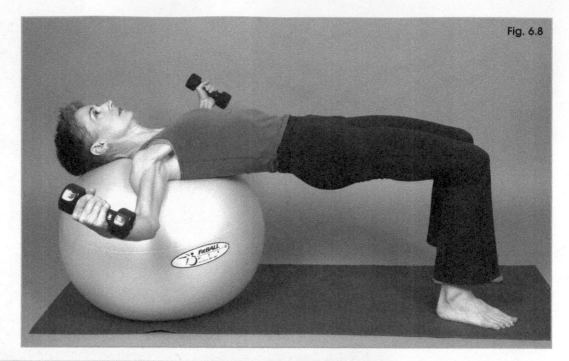

Fig. 6.8

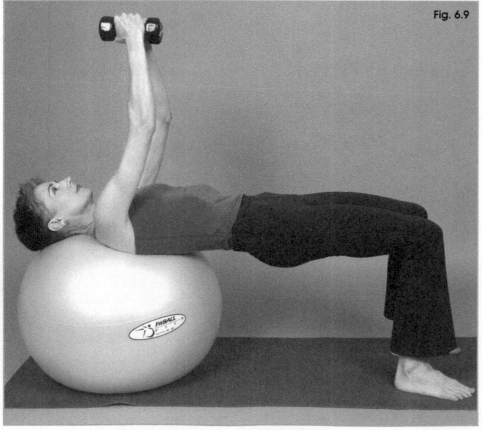

Fig. 6.9

movement 3: flies

1. Open your arms to the sides, keeping the elbows slightly bent. Hug the ball with the back of your upper arms **(fig. 6.8)**.

2. Keeping your elbows slightly bent, exhale to squeeze your arms together in a large semi-circle, as if hugging a thick tree **(fig. 6.9)**.

3. Reverse the circular motion to return to the arms-open position. Repeat eight to ten times.

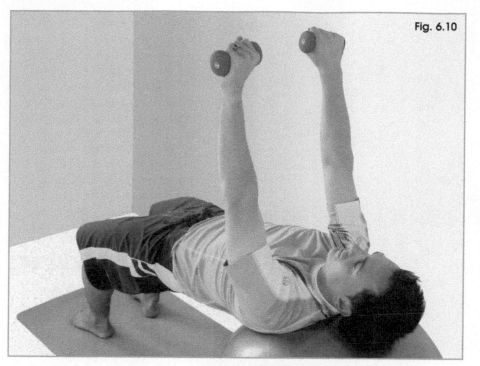

Fig. 6.10

movement 4: backstroke

1. Begin with arms above the shoulders **(fig. 6.10)**.

2. Exhale to move the arms slowly in a diagonal pattern. One arm (palm down) is lowered toward your thigh as the other (palm up) moves back toward your ear **(fig. 6.11)**.

3. Inhale to return to the start position, hands above shoulders.

4. Exhale to move the arms slowly in opposite directions.

5. Repeat eight to ten times. Remember to draw the navel toward the spine and not to let the spine arch or sag.

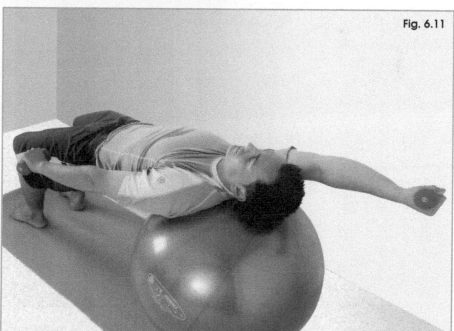

Fig. 6.11

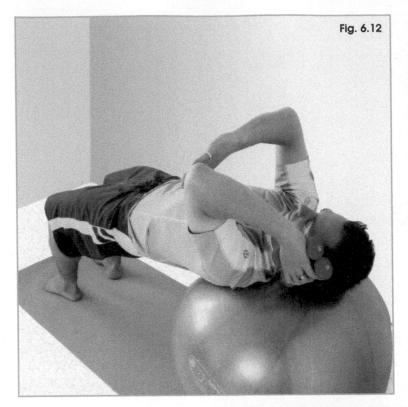

Fig. 6.12

movement 5: triceps isolator

1. Holding one or two weights in the left hand, lift the left elbow straight up toward the ceiling. Then place your right hand at the base of your left elbow, palm out, and lower your left hand toward your left ear **(fig. 612)**.

2. On the exhalation, straighten your left arm **(fig. 6.13)**. On the inhalation, slowly lower your left hand toward your right ear **(fig. 6.14)**. On the exhalation lift the weight toward the ceiling **(fig. 6.15)**.

3. Repeat eight to ten times, alternating between left and right ears.

4. Switch arms and repeat eight to ten times.

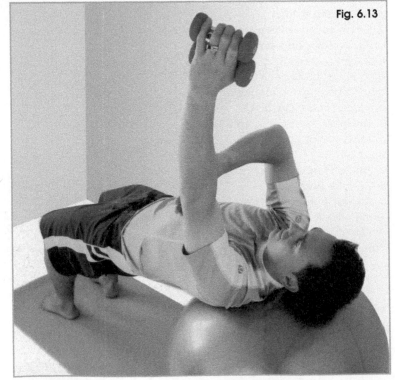

Fig. 6.13

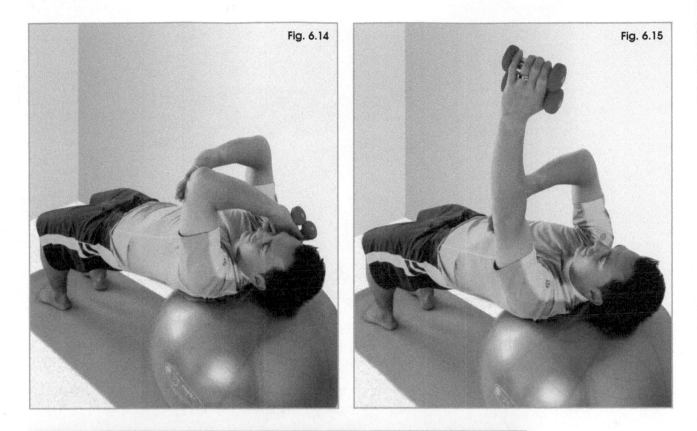

Fig. 6.14

Fig. 6.15

Safety in the Gym

- If you are doing weights on the ball in a gym you will need to wear shoes. There are too many sharp objects in a gym setting and owners will not allow bare feet.

- Always inspect a gym ball carefully before you use it.

- Make sure free weights are tightly affixed to the bar.

- If you use any machines, make sure the selector key is firmly pushed into machine and twisted so that it is locked into place.

- Do not touch cables or pulleys when they are in use.

- Children, older populations, and people with osteoporosis should avoid the use of heavy resistance equipment. Children should not be left unsupervised with heavy weights or with balls that are too big for them.

- Pain should not occur during any exercise. At the first twinge of pain, stop. If you experience dizziness or shortness of breath, discontinue exercise.

- Avoid ballistic or jerky movements. Work in good alignment.

- Do not hold your breath. Use an exhalation during the exertion stage of a movement.

- Be aware that some medications may alter how you react to exercise and weight training.

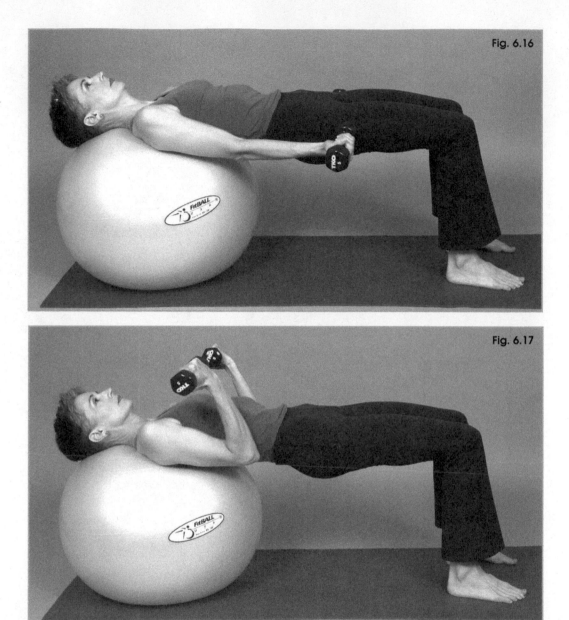

Fig. 6.16

Fig. 6.17

movement 6: bicep curls on the back

1. Hold one weight in each hand. Straighten your arms out so that they are just beside your hips. Palms are up; if possible, your elbows should not rest on the ball **(fig. 6.16)**.
2. On the exhalation bend both arms, bringing your hands toward your shoulders **(fig. 6.17)**. As you approach your

shoulders, note the point at which the biceps are no longer actively working. Stop your movement just before that point for maximal benefit to the muscle.
3. Inhale to bring the arms back toward the hips. Exhale to bend the arms.
4. Repeat eight to ten times. For variety, alternate between left and right arms for twice as many reps.

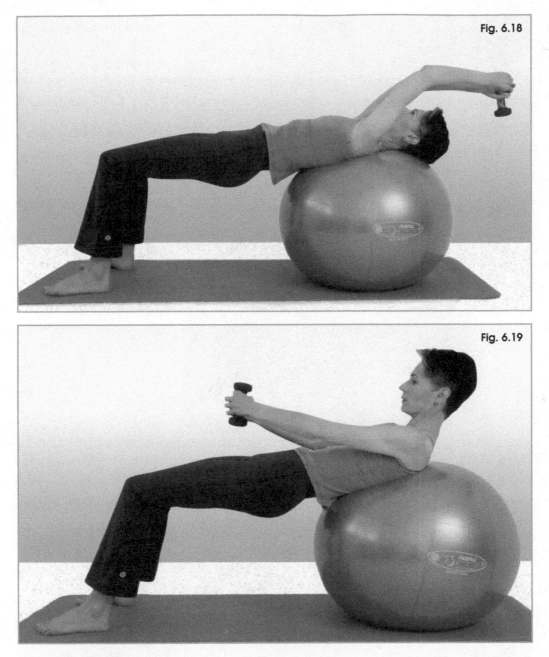

Fig. 6.18

Fig. 6.19

movement 7: pullover with abdominal curl

1. Begin by stretching the arms over-head. Using one 2-, 3-, or 5-pound weight, wrap your thumbs around the bar with one thumb resting on the other and the palms of your hands against the head of the dumbbell **(fig. 6.18)**.

2. Keeping the arms relatively straight, curl the body forward on an exhalation, bringing the weight almost to the hips **(fig. 6.19)**.

3. Inhale back. Exhale forward.

4. Repeat eight to ten times.

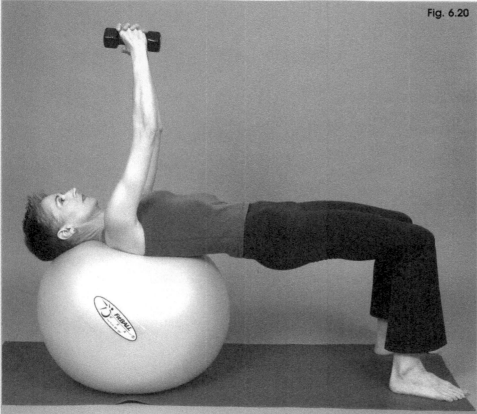

Fig. 6.20

movement 8: *from side to side*

1. Holding one weight, extend your arms over your chest **(fig. 6.20)**.

2. Keeping both arms straight, slowly roll in one direction on the exhalation. The ball will roll slightly. Twist from the abdominals, not the shoulders, keeping your vision trained on the weight. The hips stay lifted **(fig. 6.21)**.

3. On the inhalation rotate back to the start position.

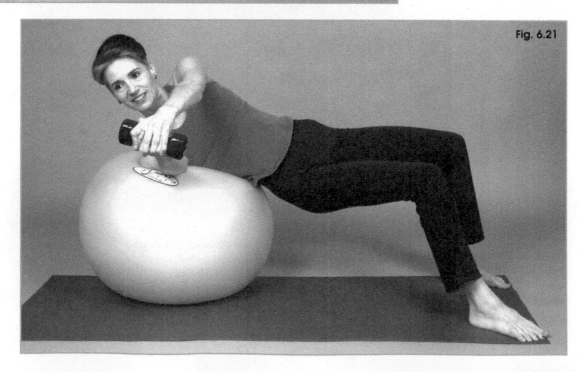

Fig. 6.21

Exhale to slowly rotate to the other side, keeping your gaze on the weight **(fig. 6.22)**.
4. Repeat six times to each side.

movement 9: modification

If your low back bothers you, curl up, bend at the hips and knees, and drop your tailbone toward the floor to come into a squat position **(fig. 6.23)**. The center of the kneecap should be lined up with the second toe but not jutting over the toes. The feet are parallel and facing forward, heels down. Most of the above exercises can be performed in this position.

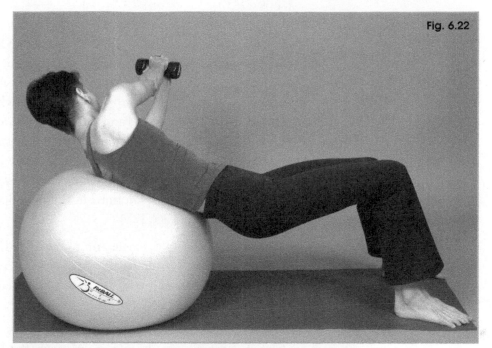

Fig. 6.22

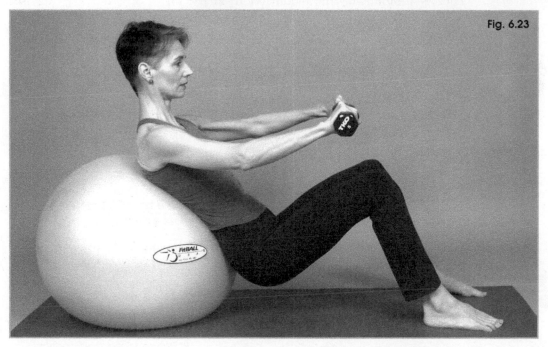

Fig. 6.23

On the Belly

Because these exercises are performed in extension on a mobile surface, the muscles across the back—the erectors and postural muscles—work as much as the arm and shoulder muscles. Keep your back straight and your abdominals pulled in as you squeeze through the upper back, pulling the elbows up and back. Keep the chin tucked and maintain a gaze focused toward the mat to stabilize the head and neck. For an added challenge, place one hand on a soggy small ball directly below the shoulder, but take care that the shoulder of the hand on the small ball doesn't creep up toward your ear: keep it down. Any of these exercises can be performed in the modification position, on the knees (see movement 6, page 128).

Purpose Movement 1, single-arm row, works the latissimus and the muscles of the shoulder. Movement 2 targets the triceps and the back extensors. Breaststroke works the trapezius and back extensors. Reverse flies work the posterior deltoid.

Watchpoints • Engage the abdominals to protect the low back. • If your low back is straining, do the modification on the knees or avoid the exercise. • Keep the movement slow and controlled. • Keep extended through the spine; the neck is long but not hyperextended. • Keep your gaze on the mat.

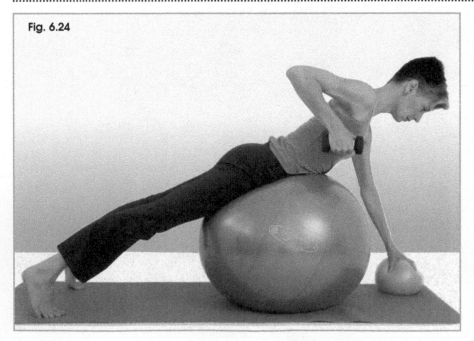

Fig. 6.24

starting position

Digging your toes into your sticky mat, place one hand on a soggy small ball or on the mat. Hold a 1-, 2-, 3-, or 5-pound weight in one hand. Pull the navel in toward the spine. Keep the spine long, the head aligned at the top of the spine. Your gaze is on the mat.

movement 1: single-arm row

1. Exhale to pull your elbow upward, lifting the weight toward your rib cage. Keep your arms close to your body (fig. 6.24).
2. Return to the start position. Keep your back straight at all times, abdominals engaged.
3. Repeat eight to ten times on one side, then switch to the other side.

movement 2: triceps targetter

1. Place one hand on a soggy small ball or on the mat. Place a 1-, 2-, 3-, or 5-pound weight in the other hand and pull the elbow upward **(fig. 6.25)**. Inhale.

2. Keeping the elbow in place, exhale to extend the arm **(fig. 6.26)**. Inhale to bend the arm. Your gaze is on the mat. Keep the upper arm stabilized in space as your elbow bends and stretches—this stabilization is necessary for working the tricep muscles of the upper arm.

3. Repeat eight to ten times, then switch arms and work the other side.

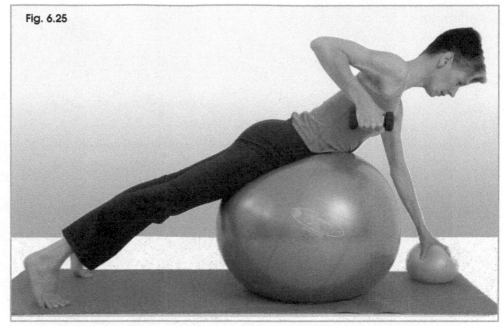

Fig. 6.25

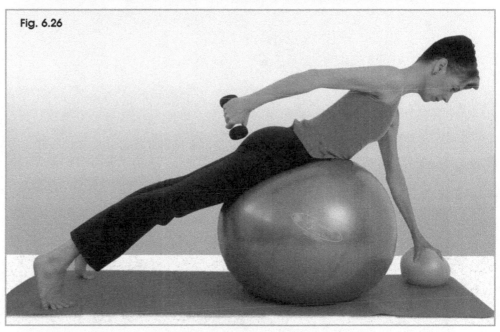

Fig. 6.26

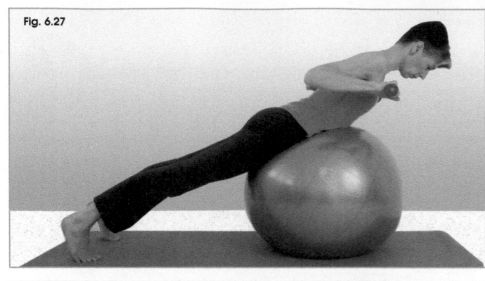

Fig. 6.27

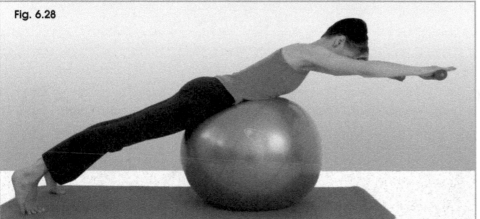

Fig. 6.28

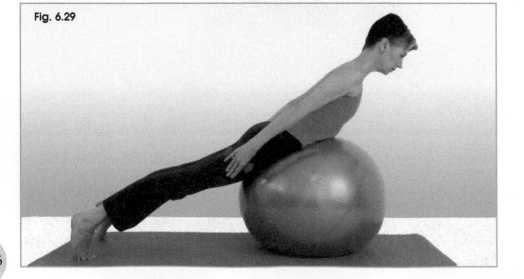

Fig. 6.29

movement 3: breaststroke

1. Start with no weight or 1-pound weights just in front of the shoulder **(fig. 6.27)**. Inhale.

2. Exhale to extend the arms straight forward, keeping shoulders down and away from the ears **(fig. 6.28)**. The gaze is on the mat.

3. Inhale to sweep your arms all the way around and back to your thighs, lifting your upper body slightly **(fig. 6.29)**. Your gaze remains on the mat.

4. Repeat five times, slow and smooth.

movement 4: reverse flies

1. Place one 1-, 2-, 3-, or 5-pound weight in each hand **(fig. 6.30)**.

2. Keeping your back straight and your arms slightly bent, lift the weights until your elbows are level with your shoulders **(fig. 6.31)**. Hold and return.

3. Repeat eight to ten times.

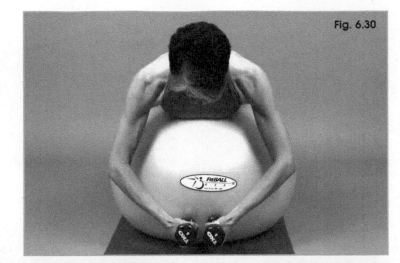

Fig. 6.30

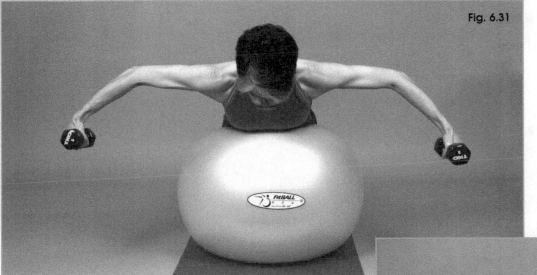

Fig. 6.31

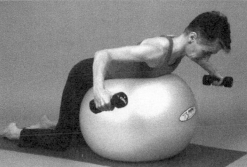

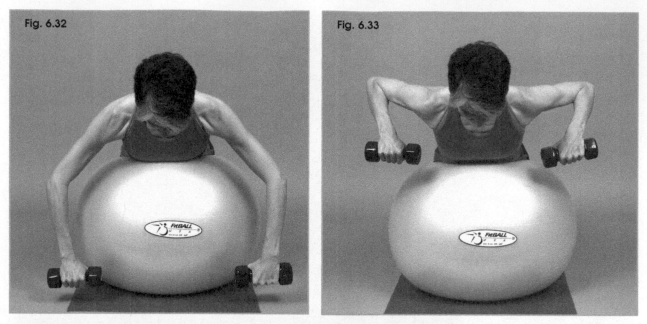

Fig. 6.32

Fig. 6.33

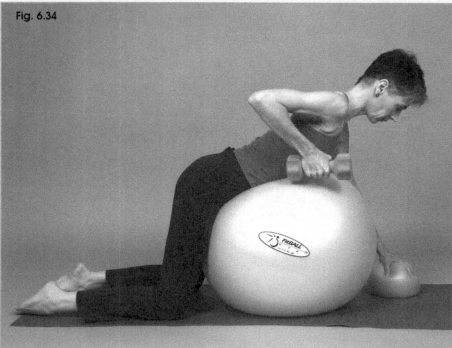

Fig. 6.34

movement 5: double-arm row

1. Place one 1-, 2-, 3-, or 5-pound weight in each hand **(fig. 6.32)**.
2. On the exhalation pull your elbows upward, lifting the weights toward your rib cage **(fig. 6.33)**.
3. Return to the start position and repeat eight to ten times.

movement 6: modification

All of the above movements can be done in this position. Kneel in front of the ball and place your belly and ribs on the ball **(fig. 6.34)**. Make sure your head stays aligned on top of your spine. For extra challenge place your supporting hand on a small ball or other unstable sur-face such as a wobble board or disk.

Bicep Curls / Wrist Curls

Bicep curls, a traditional weight-training exercise, is enhanced when you use the surface of the ball to rest your forearm and isolate the bicep. In movement 1 you can choose to use a heavier weight and focus on the eccentric contraction, when the muscle elongates under the load, as you slowly lower the weight. In movement 2 you sit back on your heels and your arm will roll on top of the ball, changing the angle of your lift. Wrist-strengthening exercises are left out of many weight-training sessions. For movements 3 and 4 you may need to switch to a 1-pound weight or start with no weight at all. If you've had a wrist fracture, get permission from your physical therapist before attempting movements 3 and 4. See the box on page 167 for another wrist exercise, this one using sandbags.

Purpose Movements 1 and 2 target the biceps. Movements 3 and 4 strengthen the forearms and wrists.

Watchpoints • Keep the movement slow and controlled. • Make sure your shoulders don't creep toward your ears. • If you have had a wrist injury, talk to your physical therapist before attempting movements 2 and 3.

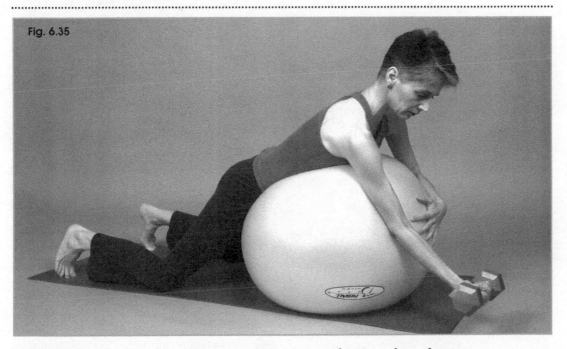

Fig. 6.35

starting position

Position yourself on your knees. Hold a 3-pound, 5-pound, or a larger weight in one hand.

movement 1: bicep curls on knees

1. Rest your upper arm on the ball. Start with the arm extended over the ball, palm up **(fig. 6.35)**.

129

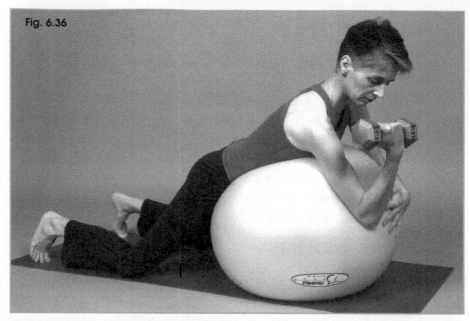

Fig. 6.36

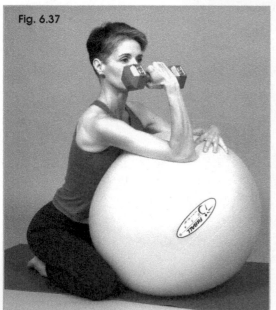

Fig. 6.37

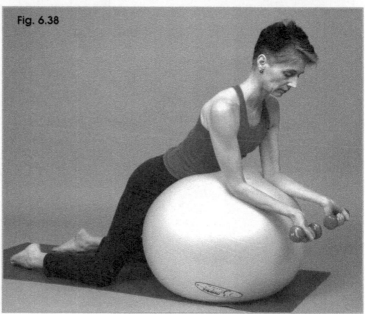

Fig. 6.38

2. On the inhalation lift the weight up toward your shoulder, stopping at the point at which the bicep is no longer actively working **(fig. 6.36)**. On the exhalation lower the weight slowly. Practice taking twice as long to lower the weight as it takes to lift it.

3. Repeat eight to ten times with one arm, then switch to the other arm.

movement 2: bicep curls on heels

1. Roll back so you are sitting with your buttocks on your heels. Your arm will now be on the top of the ball. Start with one arm extended over the ball.

2. On the exhalation curl your arm upward, keeping the upper arm still **(fig. 6.37)**.

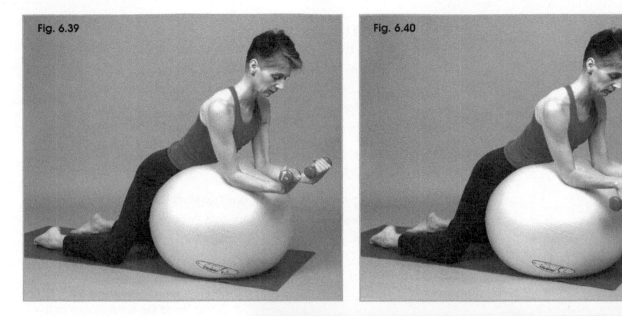

Fig. 6.39

Fig. 6.40

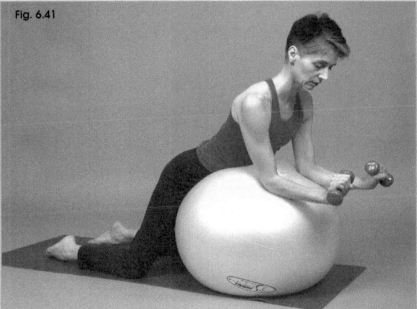

Fig. 6.41

3. Repeat eight to ten times, then change arms and repeat on the other side.

movement 3: wrist curls, palms up

1. Rest your forearms on the ball, holding no weight or a 1-pound weight in each hand. Extend your wrists **(fig. 6.38)**.

2. On the exhalation bend your wrists, pulling the weights closer to your body **(fig. 6.39)**.

3. On the inhalation lower the weights to the starting position.

4. Repeat eight to ten times.

movement 4: wrist curls, palms down

1. Work in the same position as movement 3, but now turn the forearms to rest them on the ball with the palms facing down toward the ball **(fig. 6.40)**.

2. On the exhalation lift your hand up and back. Your forearms remain supported on the ball **(fig. 6.41)**.

3. On the inhalation, lower the weights to the starting position.

4. Repeat eight to ten times.

Side-Lying Arm Work

This exercise works the support muscles of the shoulder and those muscles that link your arms to the shoulder blades and stabilize the upper arm in its socket. The position of the shoulder rotation will influence which part of the deltoid (outer shoulder muscle) is being worked. This exercise can be done on one knee or in a wide stance for extra challenge.

Purpose Movement 1 strengthens the rotator cuff muscles; movement 2 strengthens the shoulder stabilizers.

Watchpoints • Keep the pelvis stable, one hip stacked on top of the other. • The abdominals are engaged. • Make sure that your shoulder does not lift up. • Keep your wrist firm.

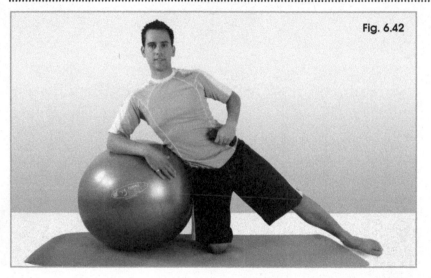

Fig. 6.42

starting position

Place the side of your rib cage on the ball and bend the knee closest to the ball. Stretch the other leg out to the side.

movement 1: shoulder rotation

1. Hold the weight on the hip of the extended leg, elbow bent **(fig. 6.42)**.
2. Inhale and exhale to rotate your forearm outward, keeping the forearm in line with your body. Keep the arm bent at 90 degrees **(fig. 6.43)**; let your elbow be supported by your hip if necessary.
3. Repeat eight to ten times.

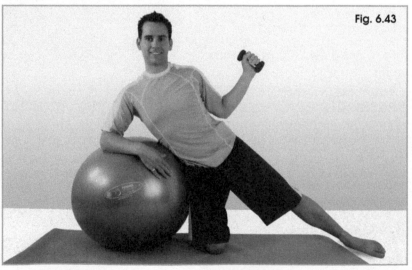

Fig. 6.43

movement 2: jab and extend

1. For extra challenge, cross your top leg to the front into a comfortable wide stance. Inhale to angle the elbow straight beside you **(fig. 6.44)**.
2. Exhale to extend the forearm to the side. Take care not to let the arm drift behind you **(fig. 6.45)**.
3. Inhale to return. Exhale to extend the arm to the side.
4. Repeat eight to ten times. Switch sides.

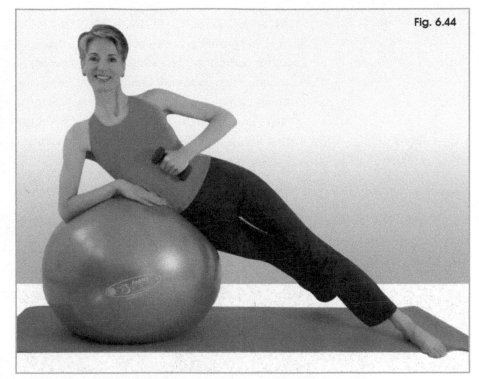

Fig. 6.44

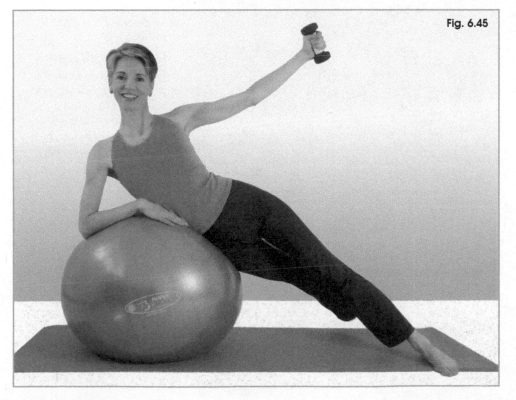

Fig. 6.45

Sitting on the Ball with Weights

In these traditional weight-training exercises, sitting on the ball builds good posture while you lift. Unlike sitting at a machine, on the ball your back and abdominal muscles are challenged to keep you upright. You can use heavier weights, but remember that you are working in conjunction with a mobile surface—so start small, then build up the poundage if desired. Placing of one foot on the small ball, as in movement 3, minimizes the base of support and makes this exercise very challenging.

Purpose Overhead press works the shoulder muscles. Side lift builds the deltoids.

Watchpoints • Ensure that your posture is good and that the spine does not arch. • Avoid locking the elbows as you straighten the arms.

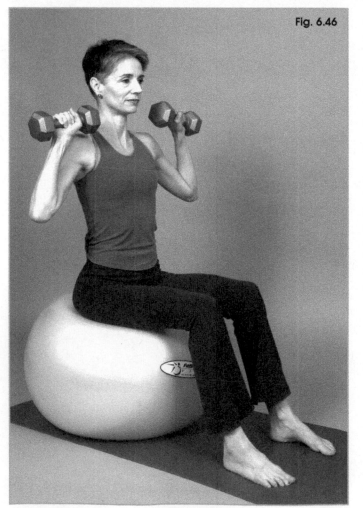

Fig. 6.46

starting position

Sit in the center of your ball. Feet are parallel and hip-distance apart. Hold one weight in each hand—use 3-, 5-. 8-, or 10-pound weights.

movement 1: overhead press

1. Begin with the weights at shoulder height just in front of your shoulders. Palms are forward **(fig. 6.46)**.
2. On the exhalation slowly straighten your arms so that the weights are just in front of your head, shoulder-distance apart. Keep weights parallel to

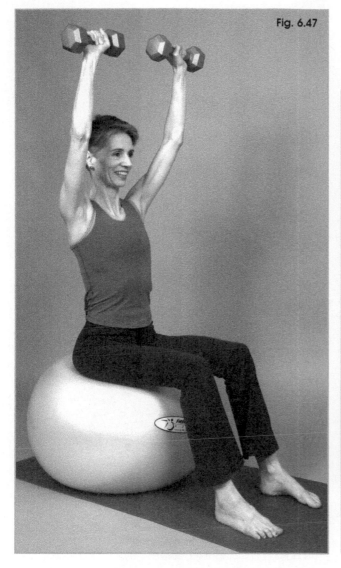

Fig. 6.47

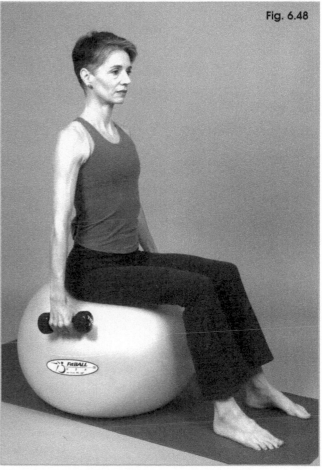

Fig. 6.48

the floor and do not lock the elbows
(fig. 6.47).
3. Repeat eight to ten times.

movement 2: side lift

1. Hold a weight in each hand by your side with your palm facing inward **(fig. 6.48)**.

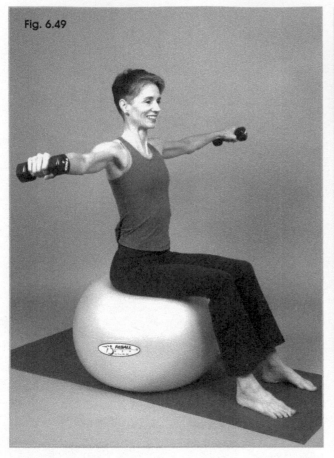

Fig. 6.49

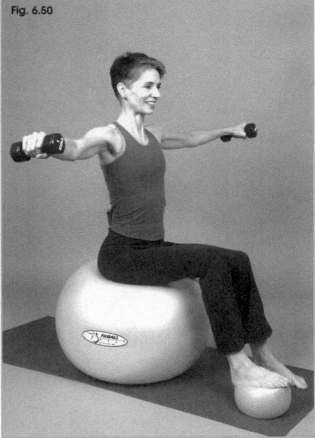

Fig. 6.50

2. On the exhalation slowly lift your arm straight out to the side no higher than shoulder level **(fig. 6.49)**.

3. Repeat eight to ten times.

movement 3: add small ball challenge

1. If desired, repeat the two moves above with one foot on an unstable surface **(fig. 6.50)**. Start with small weights and build up in weight if desired.

2. Repeat eight to ten times.

Free Weights Versus Weight Machines

Whether you are using machines or free weights, when you work with weights you are providing stress for the muscles as they go through a range of motion. The more you use the equipment the more you will get used to it. Ask a knowledgeable friend or hire a trainer to show you around.

There are advantages to both free weights (small barbells held in the hand) and to machines. Some machines don't allow for the same range of motion as you can get with free weights. The bar on a machine travels up and down at the same angle, whereas with free weights the motion of the lift will vary depending on the body's structure or on whether you hold the grip with the palms forward or backward or facing each other. When you hold free weights in your hands it is possible to vary the point at which the maximum resistance load is experienced by changing your position with respect to gravity. Free weights allow you to work each arm separately, as one arm is always stronger than the other. In addition, you can add one or two pounds at a time, whereas with machines the plates usually graduate in five- or ten-pound increments. Sitting at a machine and lifting a weight above your head will be experienced differently from sitting on a ball and doing the same movement. When working with free weights, you must use your own body—not the

machine—to stabilize your body and control the movement. Thus, you will be able to lift less weight with free weights than with a machine, even though the exercise may seem to be the same.

If you have a gym membership you may want to try out the weight machines, but be aware of their limitations. Because a machine takes a lot of your body's weight, beginners may find machines more pleasurable and easier than working with free weights. With weight machines you are often sitting down, and if the machines are set up correctly for you they are easy to operate. Most machines allow single-plane movement only, so it is important to add free weights to your machine exercises.

The Pilates apparatuses are especially designed to add resistance and to enhance the movements by becoming extensions of your body. The springs and pulleys of the Pilates equipment are designed to build long, lean muscles and guide the body to work as a unit. Joseph Pilates' most famous disciple, Romana Kryzanowska, makes the distinction between a Pilates apparatus and a machine. "A machine does something to you," she notes. "With the apparatus, you do the work." If you get a chance to visit a local Pilates studio and try out the apparatus, you will be in for a real treat. And you may feel more at home in a Pilates studio than in a gym setting.

When you weight train you build strength and balance. However, the stronger you become the tighter your muscles become. The next chapter will get you started on an essential stretching program and help you set relaxation into your schedule.

Some women are intimidated by the machines and barbells in a gym. The check-in below will help set straight some of the myths around weight training.

Check-In: Weight Training and Women

There are many reservations that people, especially women, have about weight training in particular and the world of the gym in general. Some women fear that their muscles will get bulky and that strength training will make them look masculine. I can assure you that this is a myth. The majority of women don't have the genetic disposition to bulk up. Perhaps you feel you are too old to begin. Remember Drs. Fiatarone and Evans' nursing-home study in which frail men and women increased their strength by an average of 175 percent. Are you concerned that when you stop training your muscles will turn into fat? Just as you cannot turn fat into muscle, you cannot turn muscle into fat. They are two completely different tissues. When people stop training completely they sometimes lose muscle and gain weight because they stop expending the same energy.

Some women, and some men, are put off by the gym culture, the image of he-men tossing around heavy weights while CNN, and many other channels, glare down from overhead televisions. Yes, a gym—especially during peak hours—can have something of a circus atmosphere. One student told me that going to a gym made her feel as though she were a teenager again at the boardwalk on the Jersey Shore. This carnival atmosphere is exactly what some people adore about a gym. Others need to frequent the gym at more quiet times or come for specialized classes held in rooms away from the action. Consider taking a Walkman to the gym and use this time as an opportunity to listen to your favorite music.

Don't make up your mind too soon against the gym. The ability to enjoy gym culture and weight lifting can be learned, and it is well worth learning.

7
Strength Versus Flexibility

My Summer Yoga Class

My summer yoga class is held each year on the same quiet oak-lined street in the lakeside town of Sandpoint, Idaho, in an old two-story house converted into a healing center. Each summer I rummage in the familiar closet under the grand old stairs for a yoga mat and find a spot in the quiet room with its dark wood trim, once someone's front-room parlor. I feel a little melancholic as I remember other summers I have spent in this town, in the street-facing room of this very house, surveying the leaf patterns through the lace curtains and listening to snatches of the other participants' conversations about their lakeside lives.

Splayed on the mat, I also remember how I despise morning exercise classes. Why? Because I am rigid as a plank in the mornings. In my body but also in my heart. Mornings are reserved exclusively for writing and, except on holidays, I do not bend on this. Just as I have not plunged my body into the dark chill of a lake for one entire year, I have not allowed my stiff-upon-waking body to take advantage of a morning workout.

The instructor, Debbie Dippre, has waist-length straight brown hair and a calm presence I associate with a particular brand of relaxation found in lakeside towns. She remembers me from the previous summers. I remember her because her yoga class focuses on very deep stretching and I am afraid of it.

Dippre, who is trained in many different types of massage and yoga thera-pies, begins the class by reading a Rumi poem celebrating the moon. "Close the language door and open the love window," the poem says. "The moon won't use the door, only the window."

In today's morning class there is an extremely youthful grandmother; her daughter, who has escaped to morning yoga from the demands of a new baby; and her daughter's four-year-old son. The son has obviously done yoga before as he is able not only to achieve the poses but accompany them with occa-sional animal noises—the Dog with a bark, the Cobra with a hiss, and the Cow with a languorous groan.

The class is small and Debbie narrows in on what is working and what is not. Thinking about the Rumi poem, one of the participants makes the con-nection between the right and the left sides of the brain, the language door being located on the left. Is this where fault-finding judgment originates too? I wonder. For when my body begins to respond to some of the yoga poses, the hypercritical side of my brain cannot be silenced. What is disconcerting is this: despite the yoga and Pilates classes I attend periodically throughout the year, my low-back problems and hip stiffness have not changed at all since last summer.

The deeper we get into the class the more obvious my problems become. I am unable to go easily from Pigeon pose, an extreme hip opener that shows any tightness in the piriformis muscle and hip flexors, directly into Downward Dog, a pose that reveals tight hamstrings and overall body fatigue. It is almost as if I am stuck in the hips—my bones are set and I can't let go. Debbie gives me modified postures to save my low back, the familiar pain there beginning to flare up. Even though yoga is a practice based on nonjudgment, each mod-ification Debbie dishes out makes me self-conscious. The well-run script in my brain kicks in: How can it be that I, an international fitness presenter and an author of various Pilates books and tapes, cannot perform many of these postures?

What is happening? Why am I in the same rut as last summer and feel as though there is no improvement in my body? The answer is simple. It's easier to continue in the way that is familiar, to focus on the exercises that come effortlessly and thus are the most pleasurable than to deal with problem or weak areas.

In my case, addressing problem areas really means stretching them out. Since beginning to focus on strength training my body has become at the same time stronger *and* tighter. Moreover, the more goal oriented I become with strength training, the more I hurry through my stretches. The body is a measuring stick of the personality. I flourish in intensity and challenge and do not have the patience for low-key, holistic activities such as stretching. The result: the tight places don't get the time they need and I am deeper in the rut than ever.

Stressful Lives, Stressed Bodies

There are many reasons for developing tightness in the muscles, the joints, and the soft tissues that cross the joints. There is a kind of pattern of behavior that people fall into day to day but also year in and year out. A sedentary lifestyle and poor postural habits may cause the joints and the fascia, tendons, and joint capsules to lose their range of motion over the years and become as unyielding as hardening cement. Body types—or rather, body personalities—create fixed patterns in the body. So do chores, responsibilities, stress, and modern living.

The six weeks leading up to my Sandpoint vacation were among the most intense I had experienced in a long time. I could not recall a time of more wakeful nights, the result not only of my workload—the sort of work hell I promised myself I would never recklessly take on again—but also anxiety as I wandered into business-related areas that I did not understand and at which my perfectionism would not let me fail. At times, consumed by the overpowering urge to run and hide, I was shackled by mental fatigue, which affects attention and decision making, and also debilitating physical fatigue. My muscles were tired, stiff, slow, and uncoordinated. I was an accident waiting to happen.

Stress, as Thomas Hanna points out, is neither good nor bad. The question is: how well do we cope with it daily? How well we cope with stress determines how we will age. That summer I thought a lot about Hanna's "red-light" and "green-light" reflexes and how they were narrowing in on my body. The innumerable responsibilities and petty routines of our lives cause us to move through our days "head first." Hanna refers to this as the "green-light reflex"—the reflex of activity and urgency. My "head first" summer consisted of fielding unrealistic deadlines and demands, maneuvering through tricky technology, and responding to endless e-mails and computer hassles. The stuff of life, to be sure—until one extra demand comes along or one rest day too many is used for catching up and that becomes the final straw that begins your life unraveling.

Hanna's other adaptive reflex, also triggered by stress, is the "red-light reflex," a protective response to fear or distressing events. As the fighting apparatus responds, muscles are contracted and readied, the jaw and head become set, adrenalin is pumped into the blood. The body is ready to fight a beast—yet when no real fight presents itself, what do we do?

Though it might not have felt like it at the time, there were no authentic foes in my life to do battle with in this time of increasing stress. Yet I would get off the phone from a charged business call or a confrontation with a contractor with my stomach churning and adrenalin pumping. Even on the days when there were no problems to deal with, fatigue and stress wore me out and I could not keep perspective. Even the thought of a complication would cause adrenalin to release. When the startle response is constantly stimulated, as mine was that summer, the results remain in the body long afterward in the form of contracted shoulders, sore neck, stiff muscles, knots in the belly, digestive and sleep problems, and fatigue.

In addition to this, many of us have been raised with the motto "work hard, play hard." In this context, to work hard means to expose ourselves to myriad stresses without complaint and then reward ourselves with hard play—exposing the body to overindulgences of food, drink, caffeine and other drugs, hyperactivity, and overwork. After exposure to hefty physical and mental stressors, rest can only do so much to restore the body to where it was before. Hanna was greatly influenced by Hans Selye, the father of stress theory. Selye's research and experiments show that exposure to physical and mental stressors leaves its mark on the body systems and uses up the limited supply of what Selye calls "adaptation energy" in the body. Another word for adaptation energy is *vitality*, and Selye warns that using it up translates directly to aging.

How do we let off steam and work off emotions and tensions before they create harmful effects on our health?

Mainstream researchers have expanded upon Selye's pioneering work, beginning to document how stress affects the body. Because chronic stress can compromise the body's immune system and lead to serious disease, more and more health plans are covering visits to relaxation and therapeutic massage clinics. Meditation and relaxation techniques are taught to corporate chiefs and employees alike to help them empty their minds and live in the present moment. Good old-fashioned deep breathing can be done under any circumstances to calm the body and focus the mind. For those who respond well to the written word, bestsellers such as the "Don't Sweat the Small Stuff" series offer practical advice for putting your business, family, or money worries into perspective.

Massage (along with other forms of bodywork) is a very practical, pleasurable way to get at tired, achy muscles and shake the body out of the rut of physical and emotional tension. During the summer of my first-degree burnout I booked a Thai yoga massage with Debbie because my low back was so problematic that it would not allow me to lie immobile on a massage table for a period of time. Thai yoga massage, an ancient therapy based on yoga, Ayurveda, and martial arts, is not a stationary massage. Practitioners move you, fully clothed and lying on a thick mat on the floor, through spinal movements and passive stretches. Kam Thye Chow, a Montreal-based practitioner and author, describes this ancient therapy, which originated in the temples of Thailand, as a "duet." Kam Thye levers the recipient's body against his own, working with gravity, breath, and directed touch to create a therapeutic dance of continuous movement.

When I came out of my Thai yoga massage everything felt lighter, every body system registered in another key. I ambled back to my motel. It was 6 P.M., slightly cooler but still hot: a ravishing, unpolluted, dry heat. I spent the rest of the evening in the local Sandpoint laundromat, writing letters at a little desk and enjoying the air conditioning (which was not set too high). The stress of the previous weeks was so far away I could hardly recall it. Exactly what had sent me rushing around my house and my city as if everything were an emergency?

Functional Flexibility

Here is the paradox: We build up our bodies to create security, esthetic attractiveness, even the unobtainable immortality, but with strength comes rigidity. Flexibility of mind and body, on the other hand, expands us, and connects us to others. In physical terms, flexibility is fundamental to the goal of functional movement and functional living.

Stretching is often overlooked in many types of training. But it is essential to learn to stretch properly to prevent injury and to give you the best performance for your sporting event. Flexibility improves your posture and lessens aches and pains of vigorous workouts and everyday life. Stretching is also a great pick-me-up that improves your outlook on life. Try the stretches detailed in this chapter when you are particularly stressed or have been working too long and see how easily they remove tension from the body and the mind.

The first two resistance-band stretches in the Single-Leg Stretch Series, parallel leg and turnout, are adapted from Pilates apparatus. The elastic quality of the band works like the springs on the equipment. Resistance bands, which should be taut but not stretched out at the start of the exercise, help combine strength training with a deep stretch in a continuous movement. In the beginning of the exercise the band provides resistance, challenging the gluteals and hamstrings as you stretch the leg out, the band increasing its resistance as it becomes more taut. Then, in the second part of the exercise, the band aids in stretching the hamstrings without pausing or freezing the body in a certain position.

These Pilates-based stretches are different from the stretches of movements

143

3, 4, and 5 and all of the ball stretches that follow. These are traditional stretches in which we hold the body in the stretch for a number of seconds, usually ranging from 20 to 60.

If you are not doing the Pilates abdominal work or weight-training exercises before stretching, be sure to take a brisk walk or do some gentle aerobic moves to raise your heart rate and warm the body.

Stretching Guidelines

*t*he more strength training you do, the more you will need to stretch. Even everyday activities like sitting and standing cause muscles to shorten over time. Muscle imbalance distorts posture and alignment, as tight muscles influence the movement of the low back, pelvis, and shoulder area and can cause lower- and upper-back strains and pain. Regular stretching will promote muscle balance and circulation and increase range of motion and relaxation.

To ensure safe stretches, make the stretches gradual. It is essential that the body is warm *before* you stretch. Never use stretching to warm up the body.

- Start with easy stretches at the point where you feel a mild tension.

- Breathe normally and hold each stretch for at least 30 seconds if possible. Use the exhalation to ease the body a fraction of an inch deeper into the stretch.

- Do not jerk or bounce the body into place. If you do, the stretch

reflex could snap into place and instruct your body to tense up as a protective response.

- Try to relax your muscles and make sure tension is not building into other parts of the body.

- Be aware of your alignment during each stretch. Adjust each stretch to suit your body and limitations.

- Understretching is better than overstretching. Your muscles, tendons, and ligaments support your body and protect your joints. Overstretching can cause areas of the body to move beyond what would be a safe range. Pregnant women should not overstretch, as they produce the hormone relaxin and can be more flexible at this time. Increased laxity in the joints increases the risk of joint injury.

- Avoid stretching if there is acute inflammation in the region and whenever you feel a sharp pain.

- Stretch as a cat does, not as exercise but as a way of maintaining your body and rewarding it with a sensation of pleasure and release.

Band and Ball Stretches

When working with resistance bands, as you are in the first exercise here, it is essential that you have a firm grip on the end of the band so it does not snap out of your hand and back into your face. When lying on your back, angle your elbows down on the mat but slightly open to release the shoulders; the wrists are firm. This position should hold the band in place. Take care when looping the band across the back of the feet. Try to maintain the full width of the band whenever possible to prevent it from digging into your hands or slipping off your feet. If the band pulls on your leg hair, wear long socks.

Resistance bands can cause injury if not used properly. I would not encourage their use with younger children. Review the safety precautions on page 53.

The second group of exercises utilizes the unique quality of the ball to enhance the stretch. The basic-level stretches on the ball isolate one major muscle or muscle group and are designed not to put the low back in a damaging position, where stress on the pelvis, the spinal ligaments, or the sciatic nerve could occur. The intermediate stretches rely on balance and some muscular strength to keep the body upright. This level of stretch is for the fit and flexible. Make sure you are warmed up before attempting any of the stretches.

Single-Leg Stretch Series

Try not to rush through the following sequence of exercises. This sequence is adapted from a Pilates Reformer exercise. Dorsiflexing, or pulling the toes back, makes the stretch more intense in the calf muscle. Keep the pelvis in neutral, meaning that you try to maintain the slight curve in the low back rather than pressing the back into the mat. Bend the opposite knee if necessary. In movement 1, keep the legs parallel through the entire exercise. In movement 2, begin with the leg turned out from the hip socket, then swivel the leg back to parallel halfway through the sequence.

Purpose To strengthen and stretch the hamstrings, inner thighs, and outside of the legs.

Watchpoints • The tailbone should remain down on the mat. • Try not to arch the back and shorten the neck. • If you feel pressure on the back of the knee, keep the knee slightly bent. • Keep the shoulders down and relaxed. • Keep the wrists firm.

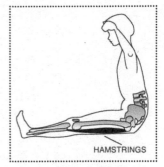

HAMSTRINGS

hamstrings

The term *hamstrings* applies to the muscle group consisting of the semimembranosus, semitendinosus, and biceps femoris. These muscles originate on the sitting bone at the bottom of the pelvis, span across the back of the leg, and attach below the knee. In athletes this muscle group may look like steel cable on the back of the legs.

When the hamstrings are too tight they can cause postural and low-back problems because they flatten the natural curve of the low back and affect the placement of the pelvis. The drawing here depicts a person who is unable to sit up tall because the hamstrings are pulling his pelvis under his body.

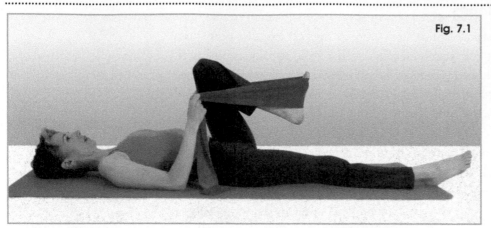

Fig. 7.1

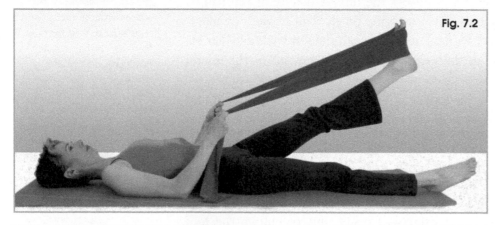

Fig. 7.2

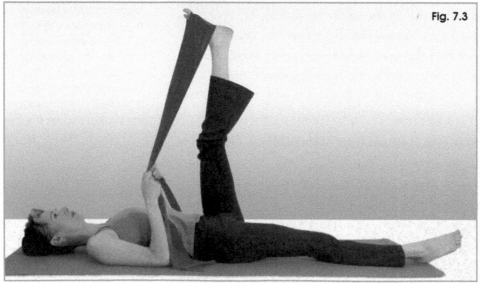

Fig. 7.3

starting position

Lie on your back. Carefully drape the resistance band widely across the bottom of the left foot. Flex the foot. Make sure you have a good grip on the band, then place the elbows down on the mat but slightly away from the body to release the shoulders. Bend the left knee. Stretch the right leg down the mat or bend it **(fig. 7.1)**.

movement 1: parallel leg

1. On the exhalation, straighten the left leg to a 45-degree angle from the mat **(fig. 7.2)**.
2. Keeping the tailbone heavy on the mat, inhale to lift the leg to almost 90 degrees, lengthening and stretching the hamstrings slightly **(fig. 7.3)**.
3. On the exhalation, go slightly deeper into the hamstring stretch.
4. Inhale to bend the leg to the starting position and repeat the sequence six times.
5. Repeat the sequence on the other leg.

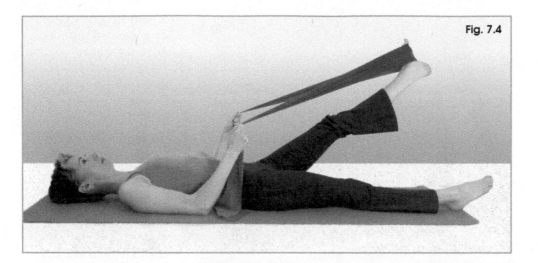

Fig. 7.4

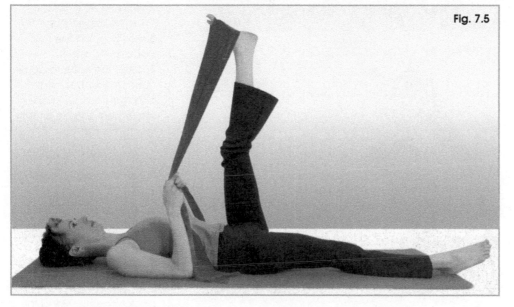

Fig. 7.5

movement 2: turnout

1. Begin in the same position as above but with the bent left leg turned out from the hip socket. On the exhalation, straighten the turned-out left leg to a 45-degree angle from the mat **(fig. 7.4)**.
2. Keeping the tailbone heavy on the mat, inhale to rotate the leg to parallel position and lift the leg to almost 90 degrees, lengthening and stretching the hamstring slightly **(fig. 7.5)**.
3. On the exhalation, go slightly deeper into the hamstring stretch.

4. To return to your starting position, lower the leg on the inhalation as you actively turn the leg out from the hip socket.
5. Repeat six times, then repeat the sequence with the right leg.

movement 3: hamstring stretch

1. Maintain the resistance band draped across the bottom of the left foot. Keeping the tailbone anchored on the mat, slowly straighten the left leg. Hold the leg directly above your hip joint. The knee may be soft **(fig. 7.6)**.

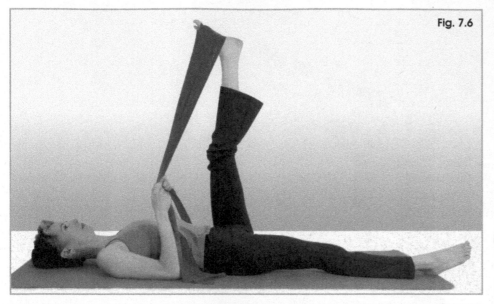

Fig. 7.6

2. Hold for 30 to 50 seconds. Breathe naturally.
3. Bend the knee to come out of the stretch and change sides. Or keep the leg up and go directly into movement 4.

movement 4: cross the midline

1. From movement 3, angle the toe of the left foot toward the right shoulder and slowly cross the left leg across the body's midline **(fig. 7.7)**.
2. Hold for 30 to 50 seconds, breathing naturally.
3. Slowly guide the foot back to the left.
4. Bend the knee to come out of the stretch and change sides. Or keep the leg up and go directly into movement 5.

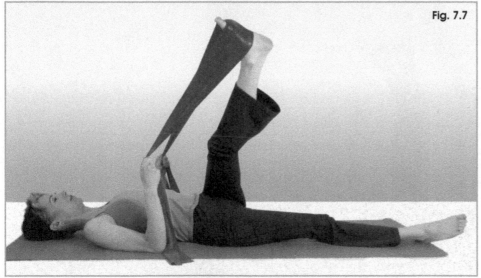

Fig. 7.7

movement 5: open the leg

1. Keeping the pelvis level, open the left leg carefully to the side **(fig. 7.8)**.
2. Hold for 30 to 50 seconds, breathing naturally.
3. Slowly guide the leg back to center. Bend the knee to come out of the stretch and change sides.
4. Repeat the hamstring stretch, crossing the midline, and opening the leg movements with the right leg.
5. To finish, bend the knee and pull the band from the foot.

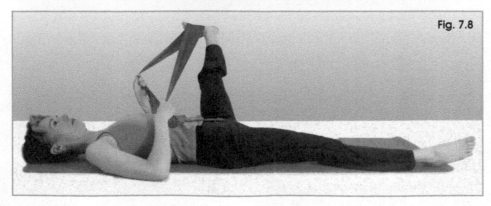

Fig. 7.8

Inner Thigh Stretch

The groin muscles, or adductors, of the inner thighs are a group of muscles whose powerful action brings the legs together. These muscles are frequently torn when they're not warmed up or stretched properly. In addition, if these muscles are not regularly stretched they pull on the pelvis and low back. In movement 1 of this series the ball supports the feet while the mat supports the back and there is no stress on the ligaments in the low back or the pelvis. Place the hands on the knees to act as a gentle weight but do not push on the knees. The amount of stretch is increased by pulling the feet closer to the pelvis. In movement 2 the small ball rests comfortably under the pelvis, relieving pressure in the low back. Ensure that the small ball is on the back of the pelvis, not in the low back. It is not necessary to hold the ball in place with your hands. Instead, relax the fingertips down on the mat and hold the stretch as long as it is comfortable.

Purpose To stretch the inner thighs.

Watchpoints • You should feel tension in the center of the groin muscle, not high up in the groin (in the tendon). • Keep the rest of the body relaxed.

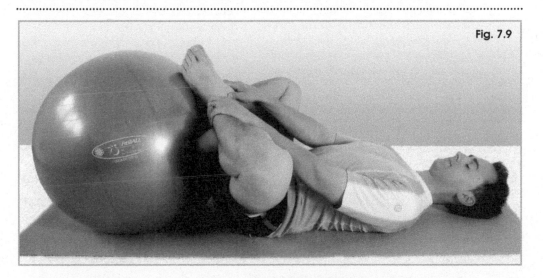

Fig. 7.9

starting position

Lie on your back with the soles of the feet together and resting on the ball. Let the knees gently open to each side.

movement 1: frog stretch

1. Relax. Allow gravity to ease open the inner thighs **(fig. 7.9)**. If desired, place your hands on your ankles.
2. Roll the ball slightly away from you and then gently pull the ankles a fraction of an inch closer to the body.
3. Stay in this stretch for as long as you like.

149

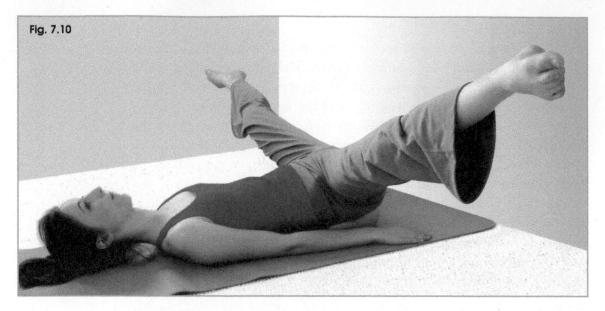

Fig. 7.10

movement 2: inner thigh stretch on small ball

1. Lie back with your feet on the mat. Lift your pelvis slightly to tuck a small ball under your pelvis (not under the curve of your low back). Bring your knees up toward your chest and then straighten your legs in the air. Make certain the ball is still well positioned under your pelvis.

2. Slowly open your legs and let them hang in this position for as long as is comfortable **(fig. 7.10)**.

3. To come out of this position, bring the knees in toward the chest and go into the next stretch.

Hip Stretch

The external hip rotators are six small muscles that cross the back of the pelvis and are responsible for turning the thigh outward. An important muscle in this group, the piriformis, originates on the front of the sacrum and inserts on the top of the thigh bone. Because of its close proximity to the sciatic nerve, the careful stretching of the piriformis is important for people with sacroiliac and low-back pain. With this exercise you will also be stretching the large buttock muscle of the crossed leg, the gluteus maximus.

Purpose To stretch the gluteus maximus and the external hip rotators.

Watchpoints • Keep the upper body and head on the mat. • Rest the back of the pelvis evenly on the mat.

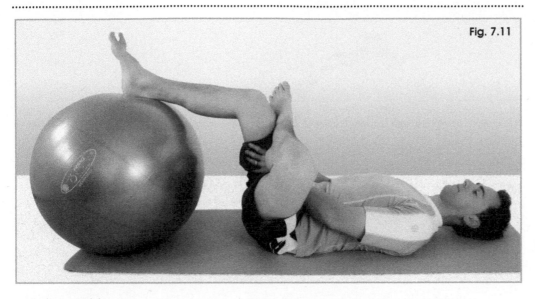

Fig. 7.11

starting position

Lie on your back with the backs of both legs resting on the ball.

movement: hip stretch

1. Allow the right foot to roll the ball straight out away from the body.
2. Cross the left foot over the right thigh. There should be no tension in the hip muscles.

3. Press the right heel on the ball, bend the right knee, and slowly pull the ball toward the body, keeping the left knee open **(fig. 7.11)**. Stop when you feel a tension in the deep hip muscles and the back of the left buttock.
4. Roll the ball back out to release tension and then slowly ease it back in.
5. Do three stretches on each side. Hold for 30 to 60 seconds each time.

Spinal Twist

This twist adds life and health to your spine. Use the abdominals to control the movement of the relaxed—hence, heavy—legs, and only lower the legs as far as you are able while still keeping the opposite shoulder down on the mat. To add an additional stretch to the abdominal obliques and the low back, turn the head to the left when the knees lower to the right and vice versa.

Purpose To gently rotate and stretch the hips and low back.

Watchpoints • Do not bring your knees too close to the mat if you have low-back pain; keep the movement small and use the abdominals to protect the back as you bring the heavy legs up through center. • Maintain the head and shoulders on the mat.

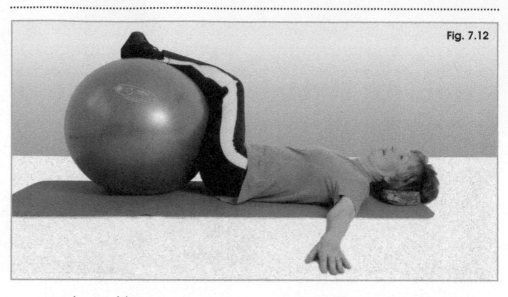

Fig. 7.12

starting position

Lie on your back with your legs up on the ball. Hug the ball in close with the back of your legs. Extend the arms in a T-shape from the shoulders.

movement: spinal twist

1. Slowly drop your knees to the right side. Make sure the left shoulder blade remains in contact with the mat. Hold and breathe **(fig. 7.12)**. To intensify the stretch, rotate the head to the left side as you drop your knees to the right.
2. To finish the movement, let the abdominals bring the heavy legs back to center. Sink the navel in toward the spine and use a deep exhale on the return to assist the abs in doing their work in lifting the legs up through center.
3. Repeat on the other side, then alternate three to five times to each side.

Hip-Flexor Stretch

The psoas is a very long, powerful, deep muscle that links the lower body with the upper body. The iliacus muscle originates from the inside of the pelvis and merges with the psoas via the same tendon to insert at the same place on the inside of the thigh bone. These muscles, called *hip flexors*, bring the thigh up to the trunk; they become tight with sitting, standing, walking, running—so many of our daily activities.

All three movements here are excellent stretches for hip flexibility. In movements 1 and 2 it's crucial that the pelvis is in the correct position to feel this stretch. To be sure that this is so, once you are in position lift yourself up and off the ball, roll the ball an inch forward, and then sink down, taking care that the pelvis is tilted backward (meaning that the sacrum is tucked under as you lunge forward). Remember—it's the front of the back hip that is being stretched in this movement. Movement 3 is good for people with knee problems.

Purpose To stretch the powerful hip-flexor muscles that lift the legs to the trunk. Movement 3 increases flexion in the hip of the bent leg and increases extension in the other hip.

Watchpoints • Do not position your knee forward of your ankle in movements 1 and 2. • Avoid movements 1 and 2 if you have knee problems—do movement 3 instead. • In movement 3, keep the extended leg parallel. Make sure it doesn't roll in or out. • Hug the bent leg in firmly to help keep the low back imprinted on the small ball.

starting position

Kneel beside the ball. Place your hands on the top of the ball.

movement 1: basic

1. Bring the left foot forward and extend the right foot out behind you, knee resting on the mat.
2. Allow the ball to roll forward to create a gentle stretch in front of the right hip. Be sure that the left knee is not jutting forward of the ankle **(fig. 7.13)**.
3. Hold for 20 to 30 seconds, using the ball for balance. Switch sides.

movement 2: intermediate

1. Position yourself as in movement 1.
2. Curl the toes of the back leg and straighten and lift the knee **(fig. 7.14)**.
3. Hold for 20 to 30 seconds. Switch sides.

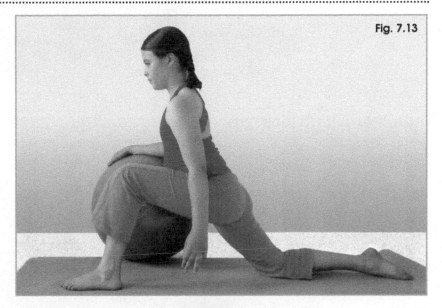

Fig. 7.13

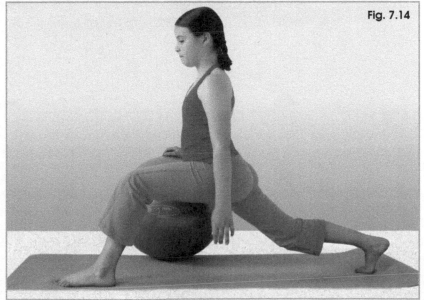

Fig. 7.14

153

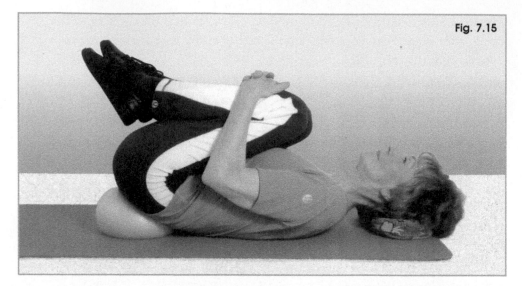

Fig. 7.15

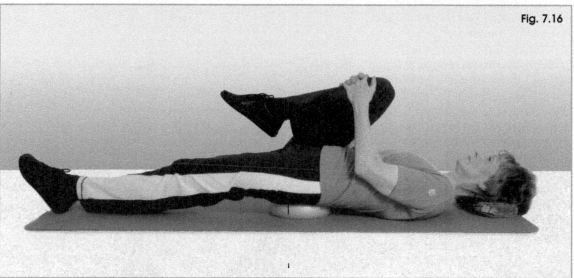

Fig. 7.16

movement 3: knee to chest

1. Lie back with your feet on the mat. Lift your pelvis slightly to tuck a small ball under your pelvis (not under the curve of your low back). Bring your knees up toward your chest. Make certain the ball is still well positioned under your pelvis **(fig. 7.15)**.

2. Holding the right knee firmly to the chest, slowly lower the left leg all the way down to the mat. Once on the mat, imagine that the left leg is very heavy, as if buried in sand **(fig. 7.16)**. Press the low back down; do not let it arch up.

3. Relax and breathe naturally. Hold for 60 seconds, then bring the left leg back to the chest.

4. Repeat this movement with the right leg.

5. To come out of this stretch, bring the knees in toward the chest and roll to one side.

Kneeling Hamstring Stretch with Ball

Touching your toes does not selectively stretch the hamstrings, despite what is seen in some exercise manuals. Besides, toe touching is deceptively easy for those with long arms. Take care when doing the Kneeling Hamstring Stretch to keep the back straight and to hinge at the hips. Hold the stretch for 30 to 60 seconds. Try to perform one of the suggested hamstring stretches every day for the health of your back, knees, and pelvis. If you have knee problems, do the modification.

Purpose To stretch the hamstrings and calf muscles.

Watchpoints • Do not hyperextend the back of the knee; keep it slightly bent for these stretches. • Lead with the breastbone; do not round the back as you go into the hamstring stretch. • If you have knee problems do movement 3.

starting position

Kneel beside your ball. Straighten your left leg in front of you but keep the back of the knee soft so as not to hyperextend it.

movement 1: calf stretch

Flex your left foot. Keeping a flat back and leading with the breastbone, slowly hinge forward from the hips **(fig. 7.17)**. You should feel a stretch in the top of the left calf muscle, not behind the knee. Hold for 20 seconds.

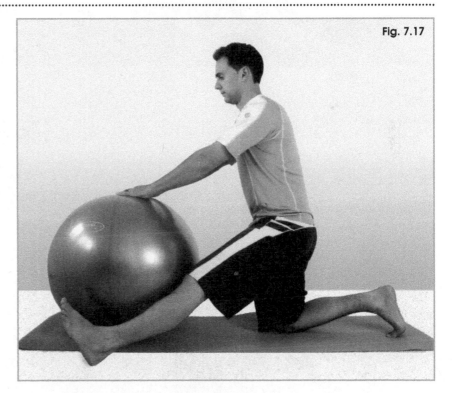

Fig. 7.17

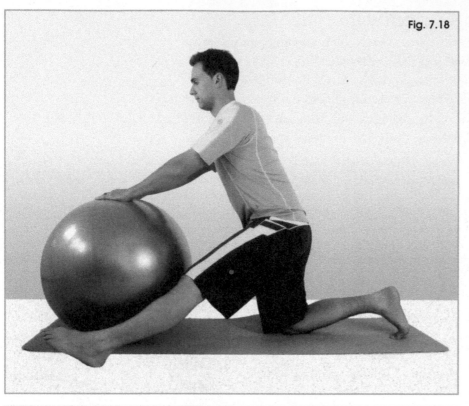

Fig. 7.18

movement 2: hamstring stretch

1. Then lengthen the foot and slowly lean a little bit deeper into the stretch **(fig. 7.18).** Do not round forward; keep the back flat. You should now feel a stretch in the hamstrings, the muscles at the back of the left thigh. Hold for 20 to 40 seconds.

2. Bring your torso back to vertical and bring one knee to meet the other knee.

3. Repeat both stretches on the other side.

movement 3: modification—sitting hamstring stretch

Sit on the ball and stretch the working leg in front of you. Wrap a resistance band or towel across the bottom of the foot. Keeping the back straight, fold forward from the hip **(fig. 7.19).**

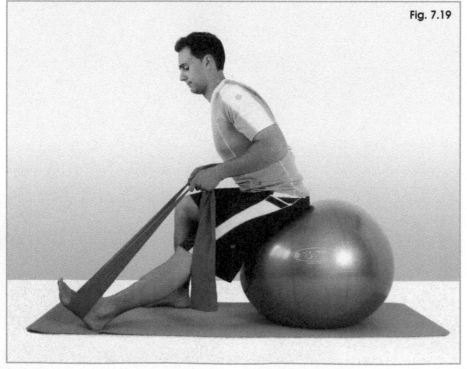

Fig. 7.19

The Tabletop and Quad Stretch

The Tabletop is great for beginners, but only if you have the balance to get into place. Notice that in movement 1, the tabletop, since the low back is not supported by the ball the small back muscles work to keep you upright as you stretch. If you have no back problems and are quite flexible, you can stretch the arms overhead and press into the feet to straighten the legs as you move the body into supported arch. In movement 3, the supported arch, the low back is supported on the ball, allowing you to stretch out the abdominals and back fully. The head should always remain in contact with the ball. To come out of the tabletop or supported arch, put your hands behind your head and immediately lift the head, chin to chest. Then, placing the hands on the ball, walk the feet toward the ball to sit upright. Beginners can review page 214 for tips on getting in and out of this position safely. Use a spotter if necessary.

Purpose To stretch the spine and torso. Movement 2 is also a quadricep (thigh) stretch.

Watchpoints • The head and neck should always be supported by the ball. • In movement 3, supported arch, watch that long hair does not get stuck under the ball.

starting position

Sit tall on the center of the ball. Feet are hip-distance apart and parallel.

movement 1: tabletop—basic/intermediate

1. Slowly walk your feet out in front of you. The ball will roll under you. Walk the feet out until the back of the neck and the head are totally supported by the ball.
2. Lift the buttocks to keep the hips in line with the knees and shoulders **(fig. 7.20)**.
3. Open the arms to a T-shape to the side. Stay here and breathe for a few counts.

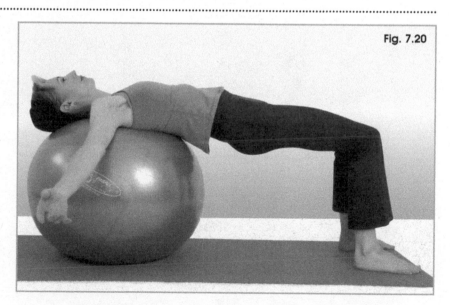

Fig. 7.20

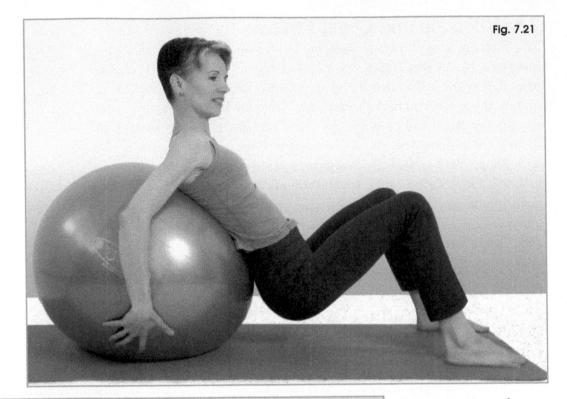

Fig. 7.21

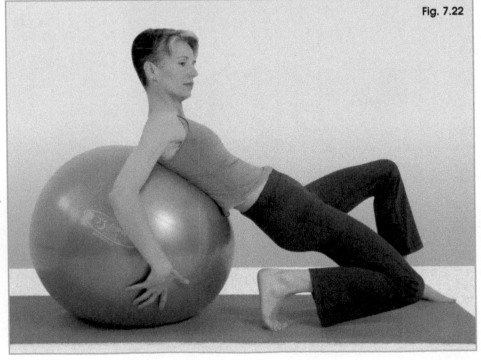

Fig. 7.22

movement 2: with quad stretch— intermediate

1. From the tabletop position, take two steps forward and sink into a deep squat position **(fig. 7.21)**. Touch fingers to the ground to aid you in balancing if needed.

2. Lift the right heel and move that foot close to the ball. Keep the right hip lifted and allow the right knee to drop. Hold for 30 seconds **(fig. 7.22)**.

3. Switch legs and repeat on the left side.

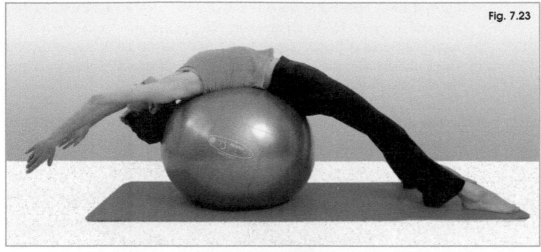

Fig. 7.23

movement 3: supported arch—intermediate

1. For a more dynamic stretch, take the arms overhead and push into the feet to arch the body over the ball. Keep the head on the ball **(fig. 7.23)**.

2. To come out of the stretch, place your hands behind your head. Lift the head chin to chest. Place your hands on the ball and walk back to sit on top of the ball **(fig. 7.24)**.

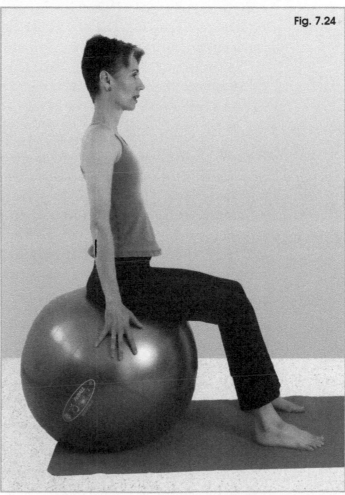

Fig. 7.24

Stress theorist Hans Selye reminds us that some stress is necessary and that responsibilities are life-long possessions. He suggests that we determine our "optimum speed of living," remembering that "occasional deviations have a virtue of their own; they equalize the wear and tear throughout the body and thereby give overworked parts time to cool down."

In the next chapter we will address rebuilding your strength after an injury or illness. The check-in below asks you specific questions to help you determine how well you are doing at fulfilling your fitness goals.

Check-In: How Are You Doing?

Goals: Look again at your long- and short-term exercise goals. Both are important, but the short-term goals are especially important, as they are the most realistic and achievable. Redraft your goals and jot down new weekly targets. Be as precise as possible. This may include number of sessions per week, number of repetitions, diet changes, and so forth.

Note where you want to be in eight months. Is it time to begin to get fit for gardening? Do you have a specific goal, such as training for a long-distance walk or a half-marathon fundraiser?

Patterns: Review the last three weeks and note any patterns that are emerging. For example, how many sessions did you miss? Were you better at attending morning rather than evening workouts or vice versa? Note the reasons for missed workouts.

Write down the specific support and resources you need to meet your goals. If possible, get the support of family and friends. Tell them what you are trying to achieve and check in with them regularly. Be realistic: are you able to continue on your own or do you need to join a class or find a workout partner?

Resolve: Are you discouraged by how hard you will have to work to see results? Many studies claim that exercise need not be vigorous to be beneficial. "The 'no pain, no gain' theory has been revoked entirely," says Neil McCartney, a professor of kinesiology at McMaster University in Canada. Dr. McCartney says that exercise does not have to be intense and it doesn't have to be done all at once. Three ten-minute walks are just as good for you as one thirty-minute walk. Three thirty- to forty-minute strength-training sessions a week are very beneficial.

Perceptions: Write down as much here as you want: How do you feel when you look in the mirror? Do you tell others your real age or do you conceal it? How do you feel about your body after weight training?

8

Rebuilding Strength

Sadie's Story—Battling a Crippler

Soon after Sadie turned sixty, she woke up one morning and could not turn on her water faucet. Her fingers felt frozen. Though mobility returned as the day wore on, the same pattern occurred the next day. Her ankles swelled up and her body was overwhelmed with weakness. Before she used to play tennis twice a week, attend aerobic classes, and go downhill skiing. Now she could not even manage her stairs at home: she had to come down one step at a time, *on her buttocks.*

After a lengthy period of false diagnoses, it was finally determined that Sadie had rheumatoid arthritis, a painful and crippling disease that has plagued millions of people over the centuries. A less common form of arthritis, rheumatoid arthritis involves the autoimmune system. Pain and swelling occur in many of the joints of the body. The disease can eventually erode the articular cartilage, the shiny whitish protective lining of the joint, as well as the ligaments within the joint capsule, leaving the joint unstable and vulnerable. Rheumatoid arthritis symptoms almost always include debilitating fatigue.

The drugs prescribed by her rheumatologist allowed Sadie to drive, have limited activity, and get to her physical therapist's office, but side effects such as fatigue took their toll. Her feet were hot, swollen, and beet red; yet she arrived at the physical therapist's office in winter boots in the middle of summer because she could not wear her own shoes. Her emotional state fluctuated between anger and dark depression. For two years Sadie used a walker; she

The secret of health and happiness lies in successful adjustment to the ever-changing conditions on this globe; the penalties for failure in this great process of adaptation are disease and unhappiness.
—Hans Selye,
The Stress of Life

eventually became comfortable using two canes, then one cane, then nothing. Still, her feet felt as though she were walking through fire. Her hands and wrists were almost as bad.

It took over two years of physical therapy and swimming exercises until Sadie was ready for a beginners Pilates group class. The first class surprised her: the one-hour class was not necessarily more vigorous than she had expected, but it was mentally as well as physically challenging. Afterward she went straight home to bed. So often in rehabilitation the therapist and patient focus on the problem—the injured shoulder, low back, knee, or painful hip. In a Pilates class, which lasts twice as long as an average physical therapy session, the whole body is utilized and for the moment the injury recedes into the background. This is a key reason why—if the student is ready for it—a restorative Pilates class can be for many a fundamental part of the healing process.

From time to time students who have come to me from physical therapists tell me something I think is worth repeating: these students will take risks in a Pilates class that they will not take with a physical therapist. Perhaps a better word than *risk* would be *responsibility*. In a beginning Pilates group class, students are no longer patients. Lying on a mat in gym clothes, they have elected to show up at a specific time and place, pay a course fee, and put their bodies through a series of flowing exercises. They must try, like everyone else in the group, to focus their minds intensely on what their bodies are doing.

Wear-and-Tear Joint Diseases

Osteoarthritis is a degeneration of the cartilage and bone at the joint. It usually develops slowly. Pain is often the result when the cartilage that provides a cushion between the bones of a joint wears down. Eventually the synovial fluid that lines the joint becomes inflamed and loses its ability to absorb shock. This can happen wherever bony surfaces meet: in the hip, knee, spine, even the fingers and toes. Forms of arthritis are associated with aging; the symptoms include joint swelling and decreased joint mobility. Weight gain and obesity affect the joints adversely. Another risk factor is a sedentary lifestyle. Weakness and inflexibility in the muscles cause joints to become less stable and place extra strain on a hip or a knee.

Small therapeutic exercises can help you increase the strength of the muscles that protect the affected joint. The worst thing that can happen if you have painful hips or knees is to do nothing, as moderate exercise maintains mobility, flexibility, and strength. Aquatic exercises and swimming in heated water are very helpful. Other treatments may include the dietary supplements glucosamine and chondroitin sulfate to relieve discomfort. Vitamins C, D, and E may offer some protection.

The momentum of the group propels them on: there is no time during the class to complain or stop the group. This scenario *only* works safely and effectively when a student is near the end of her or his rehabilitation process, in the correct level group, and with a qualified teacher who, aware of how a certain disease or injury affects the body, has devised suitable modifications of the exercises.

Sadie began to thrive on the energy and social support that the group offered and she no longer felt victimized by her pain. In fact, now attending twice and sometimes three times a week, she noticed some people in the class were worse off than her. "Over the years what I most learned about being in pain was to focus on something else, not just myself," Sadie told me. "It was a huge step up to be in a group class and to even give occasional support to others."

Rheumatoid arthritis is a serious medical problem and only so much can be done against this chronic, systemic disease. But by educating herself on the disease and taking responsibility for her health, Sadie retards the forces at work on her body, maintains function, and decreases depression and pain. Her continued mobility and improving health are certainly arguments for the benefits of taking responsibility for one's own body. Normal health, believed Joseph Pilates, is one's birthright and one's duty to not only attain but to maintain.

In *Your Health*, first published in 1934 and then reissued in 1998 by Presentation Dynamics, Joseph Pilates claims that the "old order" must be cast aside so that the benefits of his system can be appreciated. Dedicating his book to the "next generation of physicians and the association of medico-physical research," Pilates blames the modern system for present health ills and lambasts coaches, trainers, and the medical fraternity for the absence of the mind-body connection in athletic training and medicine. He named his system "Contrology," the conscious control of all muscular movements of the body by the mind. *Your Health* makes many claims, some scientifically unproven, but it is a fascinating look into Pilates' original thought processes concerning this method of training. The root of his personal philosophy and principles was that if people respect the mind-body interaction and take responsibility for their bodies they can overcome major health problems.

Thomas Hanna also believed that the somatic viewpoint—the internalized, self-sensing perception of oneself—must be added to the objective, scientific approach to appreciate fully how it is humans age and to quell many of the health problems that threaten us as a society. *Soma* is a Greek word for "living body." Hanna's somatic viewpoint complements and completes the externalized third-person view of "body" as seen by many scientists and doctors. Hanna stresses that both approaches are valid but that a somatic viewpoint inspires people to be self-aware and self-responsible.

The Science of Back Pain

Even practitioners who approach the epidemic of low-back pain from a physiological and a somatic approach can be stumped by the pain that affects nearly two-thirds of North Americans each year. Rick Jemmett, physical therapist and author, is not often stumped by pain. He presents a cutting-edge, research-based approach to low-back pain based on the Queensland, Australian, model of spinal stabilization. In the revised (second) edition of *Spinal Stabilization: The New Science of Back Pain,* Jemmett makes a distinction between prescribing exercises for those with healthy backs and prescribing for those with unhealthy backs and low-back pain. He makes this distinction because doing all the back- and abdominal-strengthening exercises in the world will not help relieve someone's low-back pain if there is a neurological inability to properly activate the key muscles necessary to keep a joint stable. According to Jemmett, this is usually the case where low-back pain is found.

The nervous system activates and controls muscles in a very specific way. The brain processes information and then sends an order signaling the muscle fibers to fire. These signals control not only the muscles responsible for big movements, such as lifting an arm or leg; they also control the small, deep muscles that stabilize the bones of the spine. Stretching, ice therapy, massage, yoga, Pilates, and other exercises will not help the source of the problem, explains Jemmett, if the nervous system fails to signal these muscles properly.

This stress on the importance of nervous-system failure and back pain initiates from the Australian research team of Carolyn Richardson and her associates. The Queensland group asserts that a person's ability to locate and hold the neurologically challenged muscle can result in a notable reduction in low-back pain. Their goal is to reprogram faulty motor-control patterns following injury. The premise of their research is that the key low-back and abdominal stabilizers (transversus abdominis, multifidus, parts of quadratus lumborum) must work together to enhance the stability in the pelvis and low back by increasing the stiffness of the lumbar spine and protecting any injured segments of the back.

Jemmett draws on research from Canada, the United States, Japan, and Australia and concludes that various muscles of the spine have different functions. The deepest layer consists of small muscles as well as ligaments that steady the spine and act as "position sensors," supplying the brain with critical information on the position of the joints of the vertebrae. The next layer is the stabilizers—deep muscles of the abdomen and the back whose function is to stabilize the low back and spine and keep them free from pain. Finally, the outer or superficial layer consists of large muscles that create powerful movements, such as flexing and extending the spine. If the deep-layer muscles are not working properly, substitution of the outer layer muscles occurs. "Muscles that already work properly will only work harder while dysfunctional muscles remain impaired," writes Jemmett.

In Jemmett's highly accessible book, written for the layman as well as the practitioner, he concludes that in treating low-back pain it is the deep- and middle-layer stabilizers that need to be rehabilitated, not the outer layer. According to the Queensland group, patients treated in their approach are twelve times less likely than people treated in traditional ways to experience recurrent low-back pain in the first year after treatment.

If you have low-back pain it is highly recommended that you locate a physical therapist trained in the Australian method to make sure you are doing the stabilizing exercises correctly. Introduced in chapter 3, stabilizing exercises are

Knee Problems and Women

Since the pelvis is built for childbirth, hip width in women affects the position of the femurs in their sockets; thus, hip width ultimately affects the knees. The position of the legs, as well as laxity of the ligaments, sets up women to experience problems with knocking knees. The knee joints will then receive considerable everyday stress. The medial collateral ligament on the inside of the knee becomes overstretched if the knees are constantly collapsing toward one another. In addition to knee problems, when bending and straightening of the knee is poorly controlled, the lower legs and feet take the shock: the ankles roll in, certain muscles on the bottom of the feet are compromised, and overall wear and tear is felt.

Another problem that typically affects women occurs when the knees lock back into extension. Looked at from the side it appears as if the leg is slightly flexed in the wrong direction. Take care in all knee bends that you align the center of the kneecap with the second toe and work on straightening the leg without locking it or overextending it into place. Strengthen the muscles above the kneecap, especially the medial vastae of the quadriceps, which help pull the kneecap into its correct position.

not strength moves as you know them. These are small, gentle, and precise exercises, more mentally than physically challenging, designed to help you locate and target the transversus abdominis and the pelvic floor. Because the contraction is subtle—think dimmer switch, not floodlight—a professional will be able to ensure you can find the deep abdominal–pelvic-floor connection and that you can learn to activate these muscles while breathing naturally and not with any other muscles helping.

A trained practitioner will also be able to palpate the lumbar multifidus, small bands of deep muscles passing from vertebra to vertebra in the low back. According to Jemmett's book, as rapidly as twenty-four hours following a single spinal-joint injury the multifidus muscle on the same side as the injured joint will shrink by 25 percent. What this means, explains Jemmett, is that just when the spine needs it the most, the muscle that would normally supply extra support becomes sluggish.

If you don't suffer from low-back pain then the multifidus-transversus contraction is not something you need to worry about. However, if you do have chronic low-back pain, stabilizing exercises that are designed to establish control of both transversus abdominis and multifidus are essential in the fight to prevent and heal that pain.

Extreme Sports and Weekend Warriors

Once every six weeks William determined to make up for all the missed opportunities. Red-faced, body soaked with sweat, he raced his bike along dirt trails and up the highest hills he could find. If he couldn't get outside he went to a gym with a rock-climbing wall, pushing himself even harder because he was indoors and "protected" from the elements. When William finally injured his knee he found it intolerable to slow down long enough to allow his knee to heal properly.

According to Dr. Robert S. Gotlin of Beth Israel Medical Center in New York City, knee pain is catching up to back pain as the number one sports ailment. Pushing the knees too hard can lead to osteoarthritis of the knee, torn ligaments, and pain. Dr. Gotlin recommends icing the knee with ice packs twice a day for five minutes at a time: five minutes on and five minutes off for a total of fifteen minutes with the ice on. Two days later, patients can add heat. Sometimes, as in William's case, the pain is so severe that anti-inflammatory drugs are recommended.

Movement is necessary to the rehabilitation process, but what happens when healing is interrupted too quickly and by too much movement? William's knee had to be repaired, which meant that he needed to do specialized exercises designed for proper tracking of the kneecap. Building up the muscles above the kneecap—especially the medial vastae of the quadriceps, which help pull the kneecap into the correct position—is a slow process. Most people when they begin to feel better return to normal activity too soon. If you scrape away a scar before it has healed, however, you will put yourself back at square one.

Once healed, athletes and weekend warriors alike need to follow a safe and balanced fitness program for life to avoid reinjurying the body. Frequent visits to physical therapists and personal trainers ensure correct motor patterns are utilized and that one muscle is not substituted for another. It may be easier to relearn simple activities, such as working the knee in correct knee-foot alignment, and much harder to alter the habits and attitudes that drive people too far too fast.

The Resistance-Band Exercises

The Pilates equipment has had a long association with physical therapy. Resistance bands have also been used in shoulder, knee, and hip therapy to rehabilitate the body while working in functional patterns. Like the springs of a

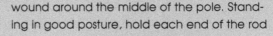

Sandbags or Beanbags for Wrists and Arms

Sandbags or beanbags are often found in a Pilates studio. Their purpose is to strengthen the wrists, tone the arms, and stabilize the shoulder and elbow muscles. You can make your own sandbag using a thick pole and an 8-inch-square cloth bag.

Secure a 4- to 5-foot cord to a 14-inch pole by drilling a hole through the middle of the pole or stapling the rope to the pole. Fill a cloth bag with two or three pounds of sand or dried beans. Begin the exercise with the cord wound around the middle of the pole. Standing in good posture, hold each end of the rod and extend your arms in front of you, knuckles on top. Keeping your shoulders down, maintain the pole parallel to the floor and just below shoulder level. Using an alternating wrist movement and moving one hand at a time, slowly lower the sandbag or beanbag. Breathe naturally and go only as far as is comfortable for you. To reverse, turn the pole so that the cord winds around the pole and the sandbag lifts.

Pilates apparatus, the level of the resistance increases as the band is stretched. And just as the Pilates springs vary in degree of stiffness, the thickness of the band affects the level of resistance.

Maintain the full width of the band whenever possible to prevent the band from digging in to your hands or slipping off your feet. The resistance band should be taut but not too stretched out when you begin. Hold the band so that you have a firm grip on it and keep your wrists firm—avoid pulling your fists up toward you, creating a crease or break in the top of the wrists. Take care when looping the band across the back of the feet that the band does not accidently fly back into your face. Inspect your band for nicks and make sure you have the correct resistance for your level. If you are quite strong, use a heavier grade of band; if you overstress a lighter resistance, the band could break.

Remember that a Pilates approach to rebuilding strength means that we are initiating movement from the powerhouse, the center of the body, to ensure that there are no undue stresses on the low back. So before each and every exercise we gently draw the navel toward the spine to activate the stabilizers and protect the low back. When the abdominal core is strong we can safely and effectively perform movements of the legs and arms.

Sitting on the Ball: Upper Body

The ball ensures that the body is in good posture, but these exercises could be done sitting on a chair. Keep the abdominals engaged and the wrists firm; avoid pulling your fists up toward you so that there is a crease or break in the top of your wrist. Always keep some tension on the band and stretch the band slowly and smoothly. To increase the difficulty level you could close your eyes, narrow the base of support, raise one foot slightly off the floor, or place one foot on an unstable surface such as a soggy small ball.

Purpose Movement 1 strengthens the muscles that externally rotate the arm. Movement 2 strengthens the shoulder stabilizers; movement 3 strengthens the triceps.

Watchpoints • Do not allow wrists to move or "break" their form. • Keep the band taut and make sure you have a good grip on the band so that it does not snap out. • Keep your abdominals engaged.

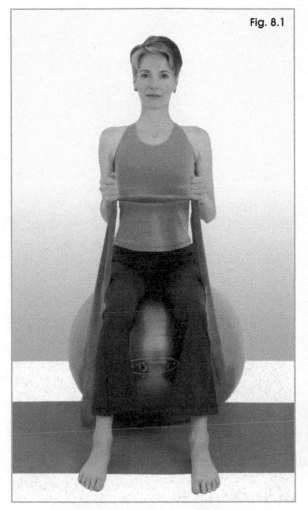

Fig. 8.1

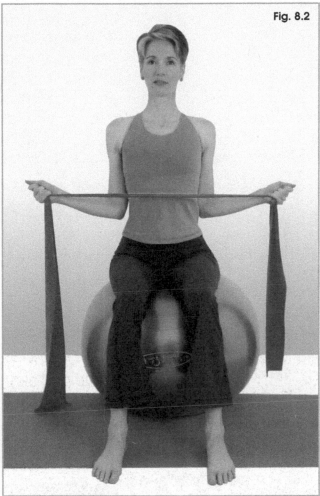

Fig. 8.2

starting position

Sit tall on the center of the ball. Feet are hip-distance apart and parallel. Grasp the band with your hands, palms facing each other. Start with the band taut. Bend the elbows to 90 degrees **(fig. 8.1)**.

movement 1: external rotation

1. On the exhalation, rotate the upper arm outward. Do not extend the elbows. Palms face each other **(fig. 8.2)**.
2. Inhale to return to the start position. Make sure the band remains taut.
3. Repeat eight to ten times.

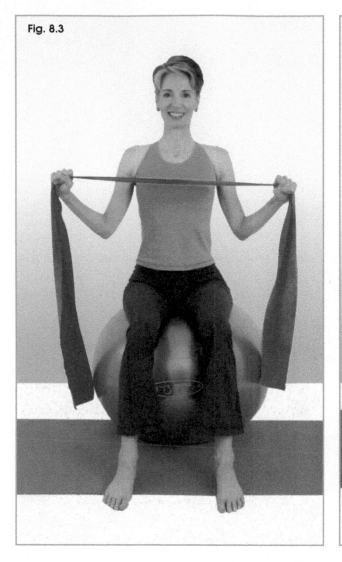

Fig. 8.3

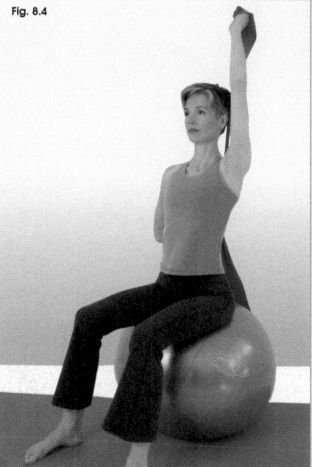

Fig. 8.4

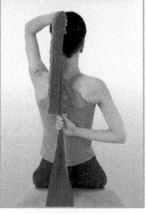

movement 2: arm pull

1. Hold the band a little wider than shoulder-distance apart at chest level. Inhale to pull the arms apart **(fig. 8.3)**.
2. Exhale to return to the start position. Make sure the band remains taut.
3. Repeat eight to ten times.

movement 3: triceps

1. Sitting as tall as possible, clasp the band with one hand overhead and the other hand firmly placed in the small of the back.
2. On the exhalation extend the upper arm, keeping the wrist firm **(fig. 8.4)**.
3. Inhale to return to the starting position.
4. Repeat eight to ten times and change to the other arm.

On the Mat: Lower Body

The movements in this series can be done in a small range of motion, meaning that if you are recovering from a knee injury you don't have to straighten the knee the entire way. The arms do not move in these lower body exercises. Keep the elbows down on the mat, slightly out from the body, and keep the wrists firm. Ensure that you have a good grip on the band. Maintain a stable torso with the abdominals contracted. In the bend-and-stretch movements the head can come up as you press the feet into the band and extend the legs—but don't roll the tailbone up. Keep the sacrum heavy on the mat. Start with the band taut in all movements.

Purpose Movements 1 and 2 work the hamstrings, gluteus maximus, and abdominals. Movement 3 works the often-neglected muscles that turn the leg inward at the hip. Movement 4 works the muscles on the side of the leg and hip.

Watchpoints • Keep shoulders stabilized and the back of the neck released. • Place your head on a flat cushion if necessary. • If you have neck tension, keep your head down on the mat. In movement 3, turn in from the hips, not from the ankles or knees. • In all movements, keep the pelvis in neutral unless you are not strong enough to do so—in this case slightly imprint the low back on the mat.

starting position

Lie on your back with the band widely across the bottom of the right foot. Angle your arms down and slightly open them. The elbows stay firmly on the mat. Hold the band securely and keep the wrists firm.

movement 1: single-leg bend and stretch

1. With the band widely across the bottom of the right foot, straighten the left leg down the mat **(fig. 8.5)**.

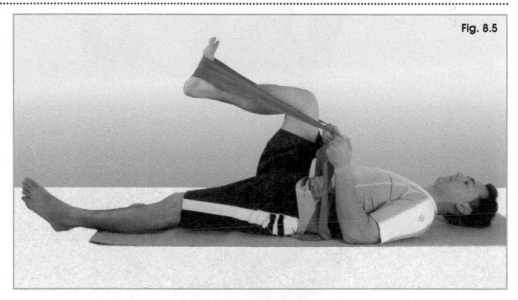

Fig. 8.5

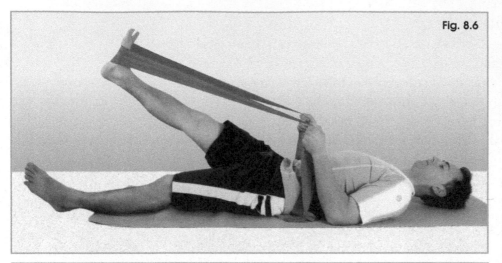

Fig. 8.6

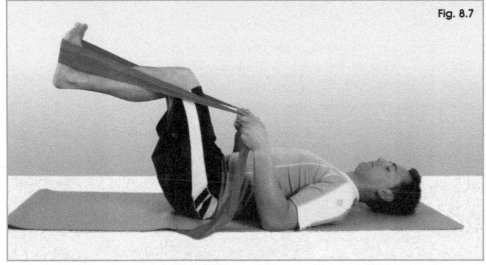

Fig. 8.7

Fig. 8.8

2. On the exhalation, slowly extend the right leg, pressing the foot into the band **(fig. 8.6)**.

3. Repeat six to ten times and switch sides.

movement 2: double-leg bend and stretch (parallel)

1. Bend both knees into the chest and place the band widely across the bottom of both feet. Flex the feet, pulling the toes back **(fig. 8.7)**.

2. On the exhalation, slowly extend both legs to a 45-degree angle or slightly higher from the mat. Keep the legs parallel, kneecaps toward the ceiling. If desired, lift the head, lightly bringing the chin to the chest **(fig. 8.8)**.

3. Repeat six to ten times.

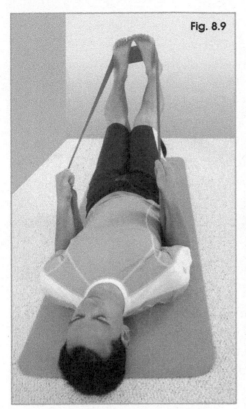

Fig. 8.9

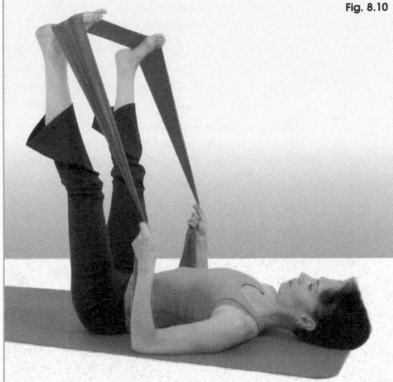

Fig. 8.10

movement 3: double-leg bend and stretch (medial rotation)

1. Bend both knees into the chest and place the band widely across the bottom of both feet. Turn the legs in from the hip sockets into a pigeon-toed position, knees close to or touching one another. Flex the feet.

2. On the exhalation, slowly extend both legs to a 45-degree angle or slightly higher from the mat, keeping legs internally rotated **(fig. 8.9)**. The head can either remain on the mat or lift gently toward the chest.

3. Repeat six to ten times.

movement 4: hip abduction

1. Continue to lie on your back with the band across both feet. Lift your legs high into the air. Start with your legs hip-distance apart with the band taut.

2. On the exhalation, open the legs to shoulder distance or slightly wider **(fig. 8.10)**. Inhale to draw the legs slowly back to hip-distance apart, keeping the band taut.

3. Repeat eight to ten times.

Extensions

Extending the spine is healing and nourishing medicine for our bodies. These crucially important exercises help focus the navel-to-spine connection and develop an awareness of the shoulder blades. Do not overwork the shoulder blades: if they are already down and in place, leave them be. In movements 1 and 2 gently draw up the pelvic floor as you try and keep the buttocks as relaxed as possible. The higher you lift the body from the mat the more likely the buttocks will naturally activate, so start small. In movements 2 and 3, keep the chin tucked and maintain the focus of your gaze toward the floor to keep the back of the neck long. Movement 3 is more challenging—you will dig your toes into your sticky mat and straighten your legs as you extend the spine.

Purpose Movement 1 gently activates the abdominals. Movements 2 and 3 prevent rounded shoulders and strengthen the back extensors.

Watchpoints • For the extensions, make sure the chin is dropped and neck is long at the back. • Your gaze is on the mat. • Ensure that your navel-to-spine connection is secure to protect the low back. • Keep the buttocks as relaxed as possible for movements 1 and 2.

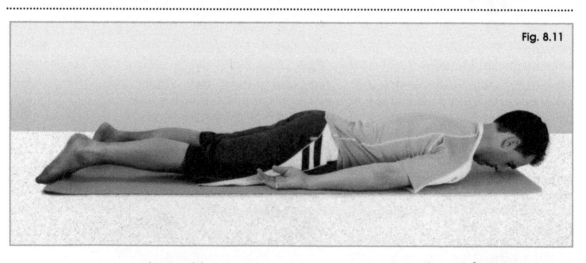

Fig. 8.11

starting position

Lie on your belly and rest your hands beside you on the mat. Your legs should be parallel and hip-distance apart.

movement 1: navel-to-spine

1. On the exhalation gently draw the navel upward. Keep the buttocks loose **(fig. 8.11)**.

2. Inhale to release the navel. Exhale to draw the navel upward. There should be no movement in the spine, pelvis, or buttocks.

3. Repeat six times.

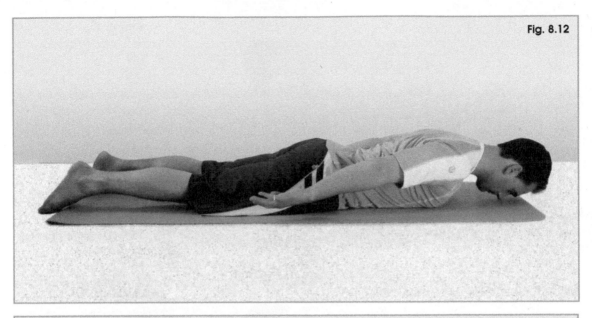

Fig. 8.12

Fig. 8.13

movement 2: breaststroke preparation on mat

1. Lie on your belly and rest your hands beside you on the mat. Your legs are parallel and hip-distance apart. The nose should be pointing down toward the mat. If necessary, use a small cushion on the forehead; relax the shoulders.

2. On the inhalation lift the shoulders off the mat, opening them and sliding them downward **(fig. 8.12)**.

3. On the exhalation, pull the navel up and lift the head two inches off the mat **(fig. 8.13)**. Tuck the chin in to release through the back of the neck. Your gaze is on the mat. The hands should be active—stretch the fingertips back, the palms facing the body.

4. On the inhalation, lengthen through the crown of the head. Exhale to return the nose to the mat and relax the shoulders.

5. Repeat six times.

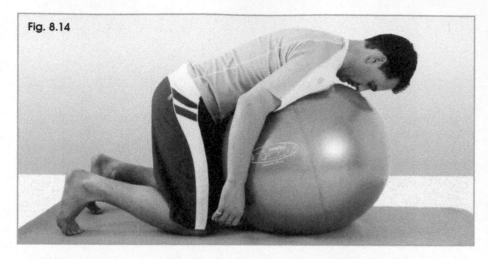

Fig. 8.14

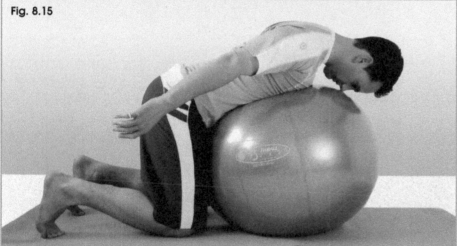

Fig. 8.15

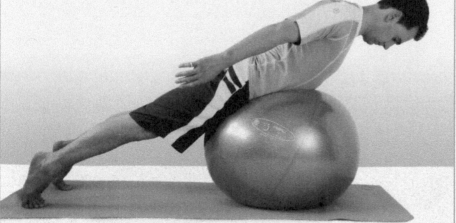

Fig. 8.16

movement 3: breaststroke preparation on ball

1. Place the front of the body over the top of the ball. Your knees are bent. Shoulders are relaxed onto the ball, nose to ball; your hands are at your sides **(fig. 8.14)**.

2. On the inhalation, leave the nose on the ball while you lift the shoulders off the ball and slide them downward **(fig. 8.15)**.

3. On the exhalation, slowly straighten the legs as you extend the spine. Toes are dug into the sticky mat, hip-distance apart; your gaze is on the mat **(fig. 8.16)**. As in movement 2, the hands should be active—stretch the fingertips back and keep palms facing the body.

4. Inhale to bend your knees and return to the starting position.

5. Repeat six times.

Roll Downs with Pull

In this next series, the elastic of the band functions in the same way the springs on a Pilates apparatus would, giving you support until your abdominals get stronger so you can slowly and smoothly perform the exercise. Engage the abdominals and pelvic floor and lead with the low back as you roll down, keeping the knees bent and feet flexed. Here is one case in which the heavier the band's resistance the easier the exercise is, as a heavier band gives more support to the body. (A band of light resistance would make the abdominals work harder.) Elbows are fairly straight, though angled down and slightly apart, so that the work is in the abdominals, not in the arms. Engage the latissimus muscles across the back to keep your shoulders down as you release the spine slowly toward the mat, placing one vertebra at a time onto the mat. In movements 2 and 3, sit on a thick book and/or bend your knees to ensure that you are sitting right up on the sitz bones.

Purpose Movement 1 adds upper-body strengthening to a roll-through-the-spine exercise. Movement 2 works the deltoids. Movement 3 stretches and strengthens the ankles.

Watchpoints • Hollow your abdominals as you come up or down. • Do not grind your chin into your chest. • Take care that shoulders release down the back. • Keep the feet flexed and knees bent.

starting position

Sit up tall on your sitz bones with your knees bent, your feet hip-distance apart. Carefully and widely wrap the resistance band across the bottom of the feet. Keep the feet flexed throughout the exercise.

movement 1: roll down with pull

1. Inhale to reach through the tips of the ears **(fig. 8.17)**.

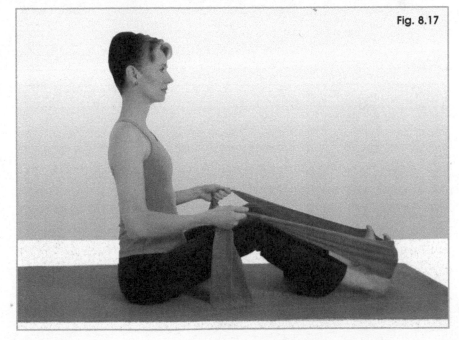

Fig. 8.17

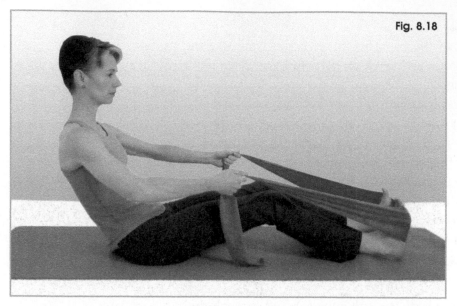

Fig. 8.18

2. Sliding the shoulders down, on the exhalation sink your navel toward your spine and roll back off your sitz bones **(fig. 8.18)**, allowing your back to curve slowly down to the mat. Elbows will bend only slightly.

3. Release the shoulder blades and then, on an inhalation, release the head onto the mat. Keeping the feet flexed, on the exhalation gently pull the resistance band **(fig. 8.19)**.

4. Inhale to release the band and exhale to curl the chin gently toward the chest and slowly roll your way up, increasing the curve in the abdominals **(fig. 8.20)**. Elbows bend on the way up.

5. Inhale to roll up tall onto the sitz bones.

6. Repeat three to five times with legs bent or straight.

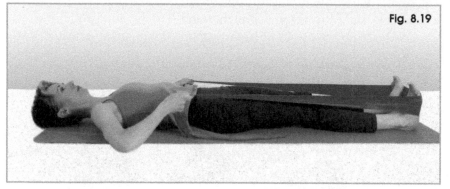

Fig. 8.19

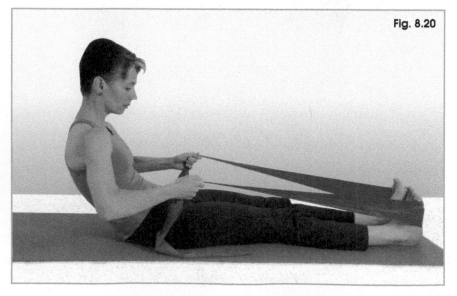

Fig. 8.20

movement 2: seated row

1. Sit tall with straight or bent legs. Use a thick book if necessary to help you sit tall on your sitz bones. Wrap the band wide across the bottom of the feet. Flex the feet at the ankles.

2. Hold the ends of the band with the elbows straight and the wrists firm, keeping arms close to the sides of the body. On the exhalation, pull the elbows back **(fig. 8.21)**.

3. Repeat eight times.

movement 3: bend and stretch ankles

1. Sit tall with the band across the balls of the feet. Bend the knees if necessary or sit on a thick book. Toes point to the ceiling **(fig. 8.22)**.

2. On the exhalation, point the toes to the floor **(fig. 8.23)**. Hold.

3. Return to the starting position. Repeat six to eight times.

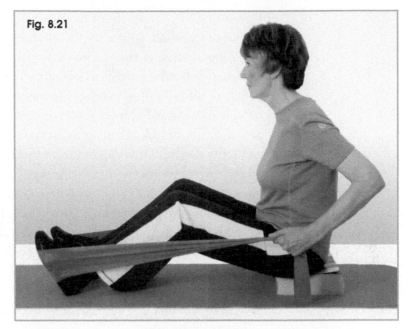

Fig. 8.21

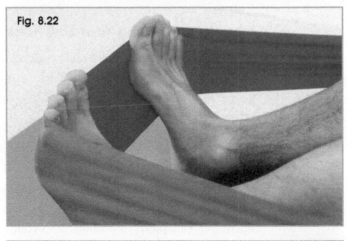

Fig. 8.22

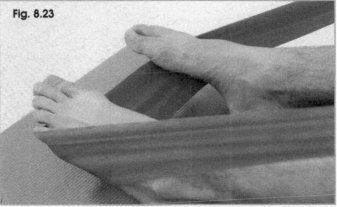

Fig. 8.23

If your shoulder throbs after a few hours in the garden or your knee aches after an active weekend, you are not alone. Chronic joint pain, including tendinitis (inflammation of the tendons), carpal tunnel syndrome (pain or tingling shooting up from the wrist or down into the hand), and forms of arthritis can plague us all from time to time. Postmenopausal women are particularly vulnerable to wear-and-tear joint diseases in the hips, knees, spine, even the fingers and toes, as lack of estrogen can create change and degeneration in bone and joint cartilage. It is important that you become an engaged participant in taking care of your joints by staying active and by strengthening the abdominal core and low back. Teach children about good back health and the importance of an active lifestyle from a young age. There is more on building strength in youth and children in the next chapter.

Back pain is the third leading cause of doctor visits by men and women in North America and the leading cause of missed workdays. The check-in below will help you determine if you need to see a physical therapist or chiropractor or whether you can ease your low-back pain with home-care options.

Check-In: Treating Your Low-Back Pain

Do you know what caused your low-back pain? Is it the result of a recent trauma, such as slipping on the ice and landing on your tailbone? Is it the result of a sports injury? overexuberant gardening? anxiety? Is the source of your pain unknown to you?

What does the pain feel like? Is it a recurring pain or did it come out of nowhere? Is the pain confined to the back, or is it accompanied by shooting pain that radiates down your leg or into your buttock? Has the pain persisted for more than three days? See your doctor if the pain is sharp and accompanied by fever or by shooting pains or numbness in your legs or arms.

Have you been diagnosed with degenerative disc disease or herniated disc? Degenerative disc disease occurs when the spinal discs "dry out"—when they lose elasticity or even develop cracks along their edges. In the case of a herniated disc, the gel-like substance between the two vertebrae protrudes and puts pressure on the nerve passing behind the disc. Leg pain and numbness in the leg or foot results. Many disc problems are made worse by repetitive, excessive flexion of the spine and by chronic bad posture. Sit-ups and other exercises involving full flexion of the spine should be avoided with disc problems, especially when acute; extension and sidebending may also exacerbate symptoms. Instead, small stabilization exercises can help pain and manage instability. Disc problems can be serious: always work with a qualified physiotherapist.

Options and Home Care for Low-Back Pain

Assess your work station. Reduce the risk of injuries from repetitive motions and poor posture by properly setting up your computer station. Computers strain the eyes and force the body into rigid postures. Keep in good, neutral posture when sitting, maintaining your low back in its natural shape. Adjust your chair and position your mouse correctly. Take care with laptops, as low screens and dim monitors cause the user to hunch over. Get up often, stretch, and rest your eyes. Try sitting on a ball from time to time. Some people use a 65-centimeter ball inflated to best fit the height of the desk. Sit with your knees and hips as close to 90 degrees as possible.

Sitting on the ball is active work for the postural muscles, so alternate between the ball and chair throughout the day. For long sitting, balls need to be pumped up firmly. Remember that a ball is a mobile surface. When reaching for a file you may slip off the ball if you're not careful. If you straighten up to lean across your desk and then sit again, you may fall to the ground if in the interim the ball rolled away from under you. When you use a ball for a chair you need to build in an awareness of the ball's location.

Practice good lifting techniques at work and home. Avoid lifting loads immediately after rising from bed. When lifting heavy objects, squat down as close to the object as possible and draw the navel toward the spine before lifting. Don't lean over and pick something up with straight legs and a round spine. Bend your knees and keep your spine in neutral (straight) as you lift. When standing for prolonged periods of time, place one foot on a small stool.

Go to a physical therapist or a chiropractor and get an assessment. The practitioner may ask you about diet, lifestyle, stress, work, and hobbies. The therapist or chiropractor will explore the patterns of your pain, give you precautions for your condition, and stretch tissues that restrict motion and create faulty posture. If you have chronic low-back pain, locate someone skilled in the Australian approach to spinal stabilization to assess whether you have any nervous-system error and to help you target the proper low-back and abdominal muscles. The nervous system is designed to activate and control muscles in a very specific way. Nervous-system error occurs when the central nervous system fails to properly signal the deep stabilizing muscles. The Australian approach to low-back pain has garnered a lot of attention lately for its assertion that a person's ability to locate and activate the deep abdominal connection (pelvic floor, transversus, multifidus) can result in a notable reduction of pain.

As some types of therapeutic and resistance exercises may be more compatible than others, take this book with you to your practitioner and ask which exercises will be suitable in your rehabilitation process.

Practice sound home care. Even though heat is soothing, it is usually recommended that you reach for ice, not for heat, in treating low-back pain. Ice therapy reduces the temperature of tissues, reduces or prevents swelling, and helps control pain. Apply several times a day for fifteen minutes at a time. Other remedies include resting your back by lying down with your feet up on the ball rather than sitting on a soft couch; stretching gently—but only if it makes you feel better, not worse; sleeping on your side with a pillow between your knees or with a pillow under bent knees if you sleep on your back; making sure your bed is firm but comfortable; and rolling out of bed in a safe posture. Bring your knees into your chest and roll on your side using your hands to help you slowly come up.

Core and spine exercises. To rehabilitate your stabilizers, strengthen your core, and protect your low back, review the stabilizing exercises in chapter 3 and then add the resistance-band exercises in this chapter. Increase the intensity of resistance gradually. A strong core can alleviate and even prevent low-back pain, so review the abdominal exercises in chapter 5. Some people with low-back problems should avoid full flexion or rolling the body all the way up from the mat, which can compress the spinal discs. For others, extensions may make matters worse. Finally, find a qualified therapist, skilled in spinal stabilization, to determine whether you have nervous system error and to help you target the proper low-back and abdominal muscles. Read Rick Jemmett's highly accessible book to educate yourself about low back problems and solutions (see "Resources" on page 257).

Practice relaxation exercises and have regular massage. Learn conscious relaxing and deep-breathing techniques that can change the quality of your life. Guided imagery leads you through a process of release by visualizing appealing scenes or by metaphorically describing body systems in states of deepening relaxation. Learn to contract a part of the body voluntarily and then let it go, consciously relaxing each muscle, fiber by fiber. Relax the jaw by resting the tongue gently on the roof of the mouth, just behind the front teeth, with the jaw slightly ajar. Have massage regularly and try other forms of therapy such as shiatsu, Thai yoga massage, and body rolling.

9

Recovering Strength and Playfulness in Youth

One in Four: A Page from a Teen's Diary

I can't stop it! This pigginess! Why can't I be like other girls and eat only one or two cookies and call it quits? Jackie has shown me a way I can eat forever—cupcakes, potato chips, ice cream—the works. She always finishes with ice cream—she heard from some older girls that it was the easiest to bring up. Jackie does it for fun. I can tell by the way she talks about it. It doesn't make a pigpen of her life. I know for a fact she doesn't constantly sneak food or steal from her mom's wallet to afford her binges. She doesn't lie to her friends and make elaborate plans to get food and then get rid of it afterward.

Yesterday was a nightmare. I had to do it in a public washroom. It was filthy. I locked myself into the cubicle and pressed my fingers down my throat. I gagged but nothing happened. I had to do it three times until my stomach ran clear. And when I came out, this girl was glaring at me.

Jackie read somewhere that it makes your teeth fall out. Wow! Tonight I'm meeting R. He suspected something after last time. He told me I smelled of vomit.

Dr. Gail McVey, a scientist at the Hospital for Sick Children in Toronto, told the Toronto *Globe and Mail* that she is worried that too much focus is being put on the growing obesity trend among youth and not enough on the obsession teens have to lose weight. Her research shows that one in four girls ages twelve to eighteen is already battling an eating disorder, including binge vomiting and the overuse of laxatives.

Dr. Sue Y. S. Kimm of the University of Pittsburgh School of Medicine found another alarming trend growing among teenage girls—sluggishness. Dr. Kimm followed African-American and white girls from ages eight to eighteen and found that, as the years passed, many of the girls moved less and less. By the time they were sixteen or seventeen, 56 percent of the black girls and 31 percent of the white girls reported engaging in no physical activity at all.

Kathie was no slacker. Three months after she began binge vomiting she took up another obsession—manic physical activity. She would work out twice a day, run as often as possible, and lift heavier and heavier weights. Her mom was thrilled Kathie was working out. On the phone she informed me that Kathie had always been a "fatty" baby, but she wanted me to "turn Kathie on" to smaller weights because she believed the heavy weights were the reason Kathie had fainted twice in the gym.

Even though her mother was obsessed with Kathie, she didn't recognize the key aspects of her daughter's problems. Kathie's secret life now also included menstrual periods that had stopped dead. Menstrual interruptions affect estrogen levels and the body's ability to build bone. Parents must pay particular attention that their daughters, in puberty and even earlier, are engaged in weight-bearing activities that build bone density. Studies show that the bulk of bone strength is laid down in childhood and adolescence. If girls don't build bone density during this time, then osteoporosis can be a real threat in their later years.

Sustaining a healthy body image is already difficult for teenage girls, but it is particularly difficult for girls such as Kathie, who have well-meaning but diligent mothers who are overinvested in their daughters' changing bodies. Surrounded by the pressures of a culture that insists on the ultra lean, many girls substitute cigarettes and caffeine for food or begin to develop eating disorders rather than pleasure in physical activity. The experts agree that these problems are situated in society and the family, that they should not be placed solely on the shoulders of the teen. Parents are advised not to pressure youth to lose weight. Instead, be physically active as a family and educate children from a young age about the benefits of exercise and a healthy lifestyle. Eating disorders are serious and their consequences long lasting. They need to be handled by a highly qualified practitioner.

Out-of-Shape Kids

Children have different concerns than their older siblings. Today, obesity in children and its related health problems are at frighteningly high rates. Excess weight and inactivity set the stage for many health problems for children, including high cholesterol levels, soaring blood pressure, and type-2 diabetes, once only seen in adults. Many studies attest to the fact that sedentary, overweight kids become sedentary, overweight adults.

Why are we having this problem? In a *New York Times* article (January 20, 2004) Jane Brody reported on a national study of 6,212 children and adolescents: researchers found that on a typical day 30.3 percent of the youth surveyed eat fast food. The youngsters who ate fast food consumed 187 more calories, 9 more grams of fat, 26 more grams of sugars, and 228 more grams of sugar-sweetened drinks than the kids or teens who didn't eat fast food. And with soft-drink and snack vending machines at each school corridor, our youngsters and teens are able to satisfy their salt and sugar urges quickly.

Added to the problem of overconsumption, many kids don't even know the physically challenging games and activities once enjoyed by their parents. Summer or winter, my sister and I endlessly explored the prairies around our Calgary neighborhood on foot or on bikes. We attended a junior high school with not only a good gymnastic program but an underground running track, an "earthworm" it was called. This 100-meter dirt track, the brainstorm of the school's P.E. teacher, was dug in the early 1960s by the students themselves! How my sister, who continued to run competitively into her late twenties, and I looked forward to running around that earth-bottom track in the basement of our own school. Weeknights were spent on the streets mastering games—dodge ball, football, and softball. Weekends included soccer on the playgrounds, skating in the park, or skiing with our father in the nearby Rocky Mountains.

Today, instead of riding bikes to school kids must be driven. Instead of roaming the streets, kids watch television or play Game Boy. Liability issues have made schools remove playground and gymnastic equipment; physical education classes, once mandatory, are now some of the first "frills" to be cut in school budgets. The friendships that are forged playing games on the street teach social skills, patience with others, and how to build relationships. "Chatting" silently into a computer or screaming at a video game cannot replace structured and unstructured play. Instead of scraped knees and chins, kids are suffering strained fingers, thumbs, and wrists from repeatedly pressing buttons and joysticks.

Balls in Schools

Poor posture, whether caused by bad habits or excessive computer use, creates many spine problems, but slouching behind a desk also makes kids less able to pay attention and learn the lessons being taught in the classroom. According to the comprehensive book *Kids on the Ball*, educators in Switzerland have been using balls since 1988, when Swiss therapist Vlatka Zeller recommended balls be used in place of chairs in classrooms. The success of this initial project led to more than five thousand balls being used; the concept expanded to other parts of Europe.

Balls in classrooms can be used as a way of educating kids about their bodies. Kids can learn firsthand how bad posture rounds the back, compresses the lungs, and causes their deep spinal muscles to become "deprogrammed," or weak. They can be shown that if they slouch on the ball and let their abdominals go, guess what? The ball will drift.

Play is about having fun, and playing with balls stimulates the brain in a way that is important for growth. Bouncing on the ball creates a dynamic, low-impact cardio session that kids love. The ball cushions the body as kids

Sensory Integration Disorders and the Ball

*t*here are many uses for balls in school but they play an especially important role in the lives of kids with special needs. The authors of *Kids on the Ball* show comprehensive lesson plans and activities for kids with or without special needs working in pairs, groups, or individually. These authors, three physical educators and a physical therapist, use balls to stimulate proprioception and develop balance, rhythm, and coordination. They suggest bouncing on a ball while sounding out words, learning math, or memorizing facts, making sure the bouncing matches the rhythm of the task. They also suggest using rhymes and music to stimulate memory and sequencing skills.

The two-in-one ball, the Physio Roll, may be best for children with balance disorders or motor-skill deficiency as it has a wide base and only rolls forward and backward. This ball is also big enough for a therapist and child to sit on together.

Children with cerebral palsy can use Physio Rolls or ordinary balls to strengthen muscles and improve muscle tone. The *Kids on the Ball* authors also recommend using balls for children with sensory integrative dysfunction. This would include children with attention deficit disorder (ADD), attention deficit hyperactive disorder (ADHD), and mild forms of autism.

bounce while at the same time training the feet to absorb the impact of landing safely. When kids take weight on their hands or feet while the body is partially resting on the ball, they are bearing weight on their bones, which helps the growing bones become strong. Placing the hands or feet on the ground also assists kids in integrating sensory stimulus from the environment around them.

Hyperactive Kids and the Ball

The authors of *Kids on the Ball*—three physical educators and a physical therapist—believe that balls in classrooms can help children with attention deficit disorder (ADD) and attention deficit hyperactivity disorder (ADHD). Kids, like adults, are bombarded with stimuli in different forms every minute of the day and they take in this stimuli through their sensory systems. Most kids can filter information and decide what is important to pay attention to; however, attention-deficient children are unable to scan out extra stimuli and so they are highly distracted by everything around them. They are also hurried, hyperactive (or the opposite, hypoactive), and fidgety to the point that they can disrupt classrooms and family life. On the other side, attention-deficient children are curious, creative, and often very bright.

The inventor Thomas Edison was expelled from school for behavior that today would be classified as attention deficit hyperactivity disorder. Thom Hartmann's book *The Edison Gene* is a must-read for any parent of an ADHD child. Hartmann does not see the rash behavior and distractibility of an ADHD kid as a disorder at all. According to Hartmann, "Edison gene" children need to be schooled and scheduled differently to awaken their potential and their considerable talents. He encourages physical exercise instead of medication.

Play and exercise is important for all kids, but hyperactive kids benefit enormously from physical activity. Unless you yourself suffer from chronic hyperactivity and its destructive sidekick—impulsiveness—it is impossible to understand how energy levels (not to mention boredom attacks) can radically interfere with your child's life. I know from my own experience that physical activity before, during, and after school enabled me to sit still in school and at the lunch and dinner tables. Physical activity, and only physical activity, quieted me down long enough to listen to others and to let them finish their sentences. Exercise will not only soothe and focus your child but it has the advantage of being something that children can use to build up bruised self-esteem, so necessary at times in our young lives.

A fidgety girl can sit on a ball and pay attention to what is being said instead of slouching in her chair and daydreaming. A hyperactive boy can gently rock on a ball until he is calmed instead of being forced into a strict regime of "sitting still." I remember watching a boy of about nine fill time at the Amsterdam International Airport. In a lounge with large ball-shaped footstools he sprawled over his ball-stool, belly down, and read his comic book. Occasionally his toes moved him through all three planes in a gentle rocking motion. Later he rolled over and stretched. I watched him interact with the ball: sitting on it, lying over it, sprawling sideways and backward, keeping alert enough to read and amuse himself for well over an hour.

Strength Exercises for Children and Teens

Research shows that both boys and girls benefit from strength training in childhood and the pubescent years, but young girls must pay particular attention to building their bone density. What kind of strength-training programs are suitable for youth? Play-oriented resistance exercises are the best for keeping children engaged, as kids do not have the attention span of adults or older

Jumping, Skipping, and Bone Health

*b*ones are not just wedges of steel. They must withstand all sorts of forces and torquing. Long, narrow bones have a spongy head at both ends and a long, narrow, porous shaft that is hollow in the center. The shaft is called the diaphysis and the two ends are the epiphyses. The hollow center of the shaft contains bone marrow; blood cells are manufactured here. Cyclically bones are renewed by cells that dissolve and clear away old bone and by different cells that build new bone. Calcium and other minerals are necessary to rebuild bones. This rebuilding process takes longer for bone than for other body tissues.

Research shows that both boys and girls benefit from strength training in the childhood years as well as after puberty, but young girls must pay particular attention to building bone density. Jumping (including hopscotch) and skipping lay down strong bone necessary for quality of life years and years down the road. Researchers from the University of British Columbia, Canada, found that jumping exercises significantly build bone mass and strength in girls on the brink of puberty. Some kids did their regular exercise routines; for other kids a ten- or twelve-minute set of jumping exercises three times a week was added to the routine, increasing the intensity of the routine over the following two years. When the Canadian researchers analyzed the girls' bone mass they found 5 percent increased bone mass in the girls who jumped rope. The results were published in the *New York Times* Science Section (December 9, 2003), where the lead researcher, Dr. Heather McKay, noted the difference was the "equivalent of three to five years of postmenopausal bone loss."

teens for regimented weight work. Recently, however, more and more kids are doing weight-training programs to enhance their sports game and reduce injury. Research shows that the gains of weight training for youth are the same as for adults. Weight training also has the benefits of cardiorespiratory fitness, relaxation, and weight loss.

Safety is the primary concern when working with young people. Ensure that the area that they will be in is free of furniture and sharp corners. I read recently about a girl who broke her nose and her front teeth when bouncing on her exercise ball and crashing into a home-entertainment unit. Keep balls out of direct sunlight and away from heat sources. Balls should not be used outside; inside, they can be easily damaged by rolling over tacks or small stones. Educate children and teens to check the floor around them carefully and to remove sharp objects from their pockets and wrists before playing with the balls. Sticky yoga mats on a carpet are the best for ball-work, as are bare feet or rubber-soled shoes. Wear comfortable clothing that isn't too loose or too restrictive and watch that long hair doesn't get caught under the ball.

It is important that the ball is the correct size. Joanne Posner-Mayer's recommended ball size is 30 centimeters for children under five years of age; 45 centimeters for five years to 4'11" in height, and 55 centimeters for 5' to 5'7". Overweight children or teens or those who have very long legs may need to use a larger ball than suggested. The rule for sizing is this: when the child is sitting on the ball you want as close to a 90-degree bend at knees and hips as possible.

Weight training should not begin until a child is at least seven years old and should only be undertaken then with careful supervision. Keep the level of resistance low to avoid stressing joints or injuring a child's growing frame. Avoid weighted balls for children as they can be easily dropped or might be thrown by accident or in play. I personally would not use resistance bands with younger children—the colorful, elastic bands are too tempting to use as gigantic slingshots or for bondage play, both of which can be dangerous.

The coordinated breathing patterns we use in Pilates are difficult to teach children and younger teens, as they don't absorb information in the same way as adults. Instead, instruct them to breathe naturally and to breathe out on the exertion phase. Young people fatigue more quickly than young and middle-age adults and they overheat quicker. Keep them hydrated and encourage them to perform a thorough warmup and warm down. Skipping rope or bouncing on the ball is a good way to warm the body.

Sitting

Sitting on the ball is active work, so no child or adult will be able to sit all day on a ball. Balls in a classroom or an office are best used as a break from the chair. For long sitting, balls need to be pumped up to correct size. If balls are too soft, my experience is that kids and adults alike will slouch into them, resulting in incorrect posture. An underinflated ball, however, takes up more space on the mat and can be more stable for some. Some children will benefit from using the peanut-shaped Physio Roll. Never leave children alone with a ball that is too large for them.

Purpose To find optimal posture. To test balance. Bouncing, movement 5, automatically aligns the spine in its most efficient position and improves endurance of postural muscles.

Watchpoints • Avoid overarching the back and popping out the rib cage in sitting. • Keep the chin horizontal and the eyes level. • Make sure children are not too close to furniture or walls in case they lose their balance. • Never bend, twist, or rotate the spine while bouncing.

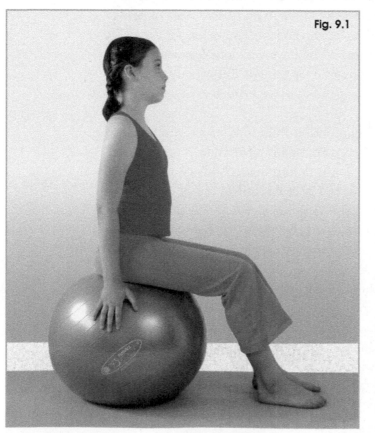

Fig. 9.1

starting position

Sit in the center of the ball, knees aligned with ankles and feet hip-distance apart. The feet are firmly planted, toes facing forward. The chin is level. Pull the navel gently toward the spine.

movement 1: sitting

1. Relax the shoulders. Let the fingertips relax toward the floor as you lengthen through the tops of the ears **(fig. 9.1)**.
2. Check your posture in a mirror or get someone to check for you. Notice if the natural curves of the spine are in place or whether you are flattening or exaggerating any of them. Sit for a number of minutes, adding time as you get stronger.
3. Think of appropriate activities to do while sitting on the ball such as watching your favorite TV show or talking to friends on the phone. If you have two balls, and there is space to do so

safely, two people could sit facing each other while tossing a smaller ball back and forth. Sitting naturally leads into bouncing or balance tests such as leg raises and toe touches.

movement 2: *leg raises*

1. Sit tall on the ball. Lift your right leg without changing your posture **(fig. 9.2)**.
2. Hold, and then return the foot to the floor.
3. Repeat with the left leg. Continue to alternate six to ten times.

movement 3: *toe touches to side*

1. Sit tall on the ball. Lift the right foot and touch the toe to the right side without changing your posture **(fig. 9.3)**.
2. Hold and then return the foot to the starting position.
3. Repeat with the left foot and alternate sides six to ten times.

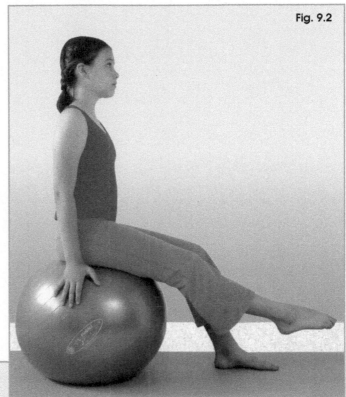

Fig. 9.2

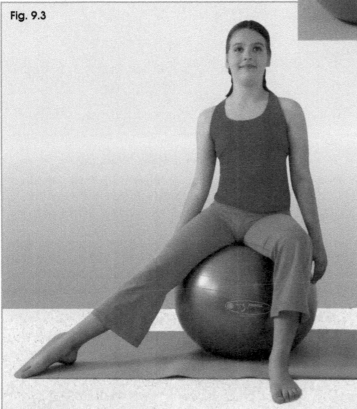

Fig. 9.3

191

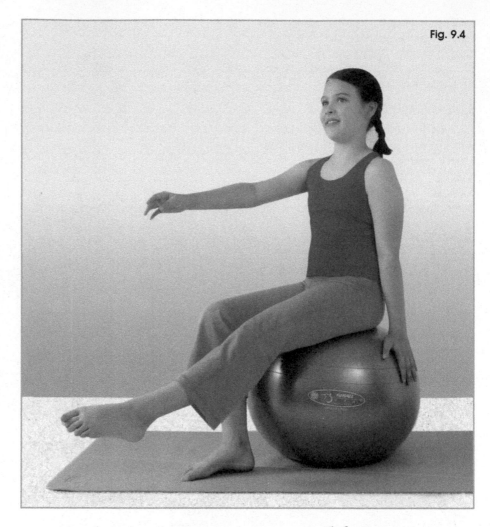

Fig. 9.4

movement 4: arm movements

1. Test balance and coordination by lifting the alternate hand and foot: first right arm and left leg **(fig. 9.4)**, then left arm and right leg. Work both sides six to ten times.

2. Now try lifting the right arm as you extend the left foot to the side.

3. Repeat with the left arm and right leg. Do the movement six to ten times on both sides.

movement 5: bouncing

1. Bring your feet back to hip-distance apart. Make sure you're sitting on the center of the ball. Press your feet to the floor, activating the thigh muscles; touch the sides of the ball and begin to bounce—slowly at first. When you feel secure, bounce more vigorously. Make sure there are no walls or pieces of furniture nearby.

2. After a few minutes, stop bouncing and sit tall. Check your feet and ankles. You should be in your neutral spine. There is a curve in the low back but not an exaggerated curve. The neck is long and the ears are aligned over the shoulders. The chin is level.

Extensions and Airplanes

Extensions on the ball strengthen not only the spine but also the back of the legs and the arms. With young spines, which haven't stopped growing, excessive arching or fast and uncontrolled extensions can lead to a situation where a disc slides forward, causing compression and pain. In a Pilates approach to extension, we keep the movements slow and the abdominals contracted while thinking of extending the spine rather than arching it. Those with low-back pain must keep this motion small and avoid movement 2, the airplane. After swan and airplane, fold the body into flexion (movement 3, shell on the ball) as a counterpose to extension.

Purpose To extend the spine. To review the navel-to-spine connection.

Watchpoints • Elongate slowly and pull the abdominals in toward the spine. • Encourage the shoulder blades to slide down the ribs and keep the back of the neck long. • In movement 3, shell on the ball, ensure that the ball is on the thighs, directly in front of the knees, before you curl up; if the ball is too high on the body, the ball will hit the arms as you curl up.

starting position

Climb on the ball and drop the full weight of your pelvis onto the ball. Dig your toes into a sticky yoga mat and be sure that your legs are straight, shoulder-distance apart. Place your index fingers and thumbs in a diamond shape on the front of the top of the ball, just below your rib cage. Open the collarbones.

movement 1: the swan

1. Plant your toes and lift your head just higher than horizontal, so there is a long line from the crown of the head to the toes. Your gaze is toward the floor **(fig. 9.5)**.

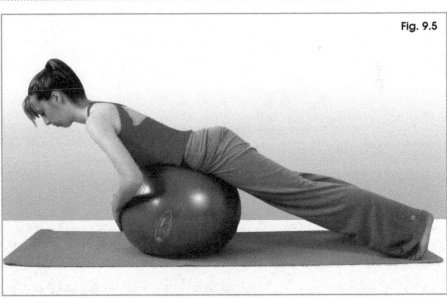

Fig. 9.5

193

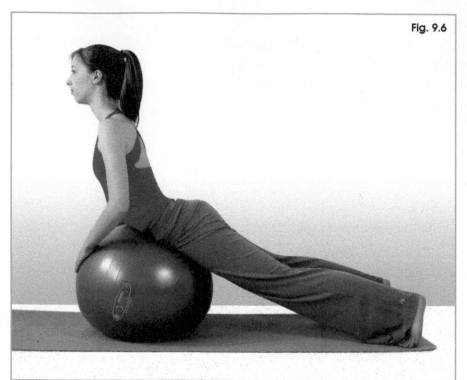

Fig. 9.6

2. Slide your shoulder blades down and engage your abdominal muscles.

3. On the exhalation slowly lift your upper body. Pause at the top of the movement. Look straight ahead of you, not at the ceiling **(fig. 9.6)**. Take 2 or 3 breaths, then slowly return to the starting position.

4. Repeat four to six times.

movement 2: airplane

1. From the starting position, dig your toes into your mat and lift your body up an inch or two, arms stretching to the side. Hold for a few counts, breathing naturally. Your gaze is toward the mat.

2. Lift one leg if you feel secure **(fig. 9.7)**.

3. Repeat three times on each side.

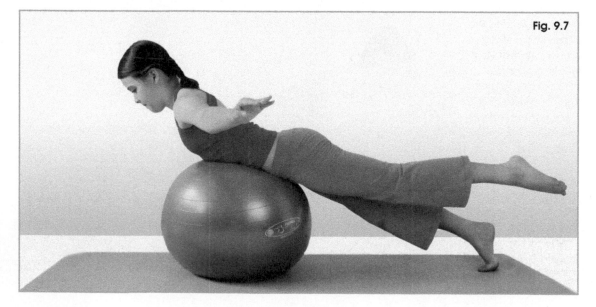

Fig. 9.7

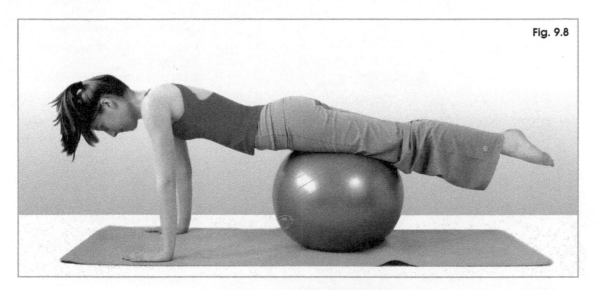

Fig. 9.8

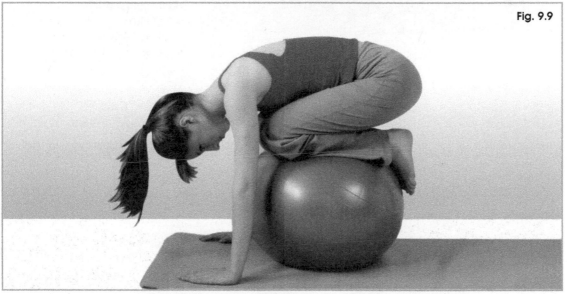

Fig. 9.9

movement 3: shell on the ball

1. Make sure the area around you is cleared of furniture. To stretch the spine out after extension, kneel in front of the ball and place your hands on the mat. Walk your hands out until the hands are directly below the shoulders and the ball is on the thighs, directly in front of the knees. This is the plank position **(fig. 9.8)**.

2. Squeeze the thighs together and pull in the abs. Slowly bend the knees and hips and let the ball roll under you, leaving the hands firmly planted where they are on the mat **(fig. 9.9)**. This is shell-on-the-ball position. Hold for a few seconds.

3. Now roll out to plank position, making sure the ball is just in front of your knees.

4. Repeat three or four times. To finish, come into plank position and then walk the hands back toward the ball until your feet are safely on the mat.

195

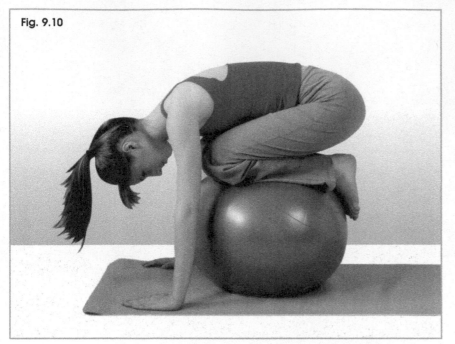

Fig. 9.10

movement 4: arabesque

1. Start in shell-on-the-ball position **(fig. 9.10)**.

2. Lift your tailbone and roll the ball a couple of inches away from the body.

3. Shift your weight slightly to the center as you lift the left knee off the ball and slowly extend it behind you. The left leg should be straight, toes long **(fig. 9.11)**. Balance here for a few seconds.

4. Now bring the left knee to meet the right one back on the ball. Return to shell-on-the-ball position and take a few breaths.

5. Repeat the same progression on the other side.

6. To finish, roll out into plank position. Walk the hands back to the ball to return to the mat.

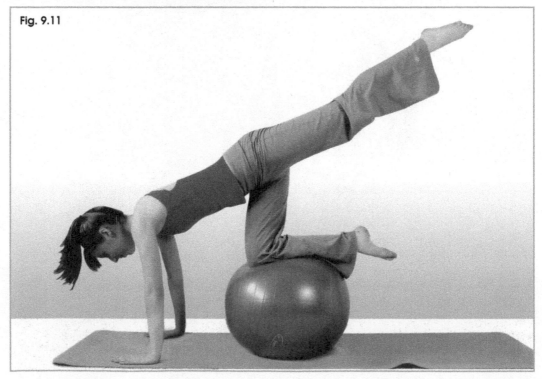

Fig. 9.11

On Elbows

Holding the body still is very challenging and works many different muscles. In movements 1 and 2 lean on the elbows with your palms down, hands firm, creating a strong base. With the legs extended behind you, be sure that your navel is lifted and that you don't overarch the back. Contracting the gluteals and abdominals will help you maintain the long bow-shaped position. Breathe normally and hold for a few seconds. Keep your gaze down to the mat so that the back of the neck is not arched.

Purpose To work the core, the back of the legs, and the upper body.

Watchpoints • Make sure the ball is not too large for you; a 30- or 45-cm ball is good for most kids and teens. • Do not overarch the back. • Keep the abdominal muscles pulled in to make a strong core. • Create a strong base with the forearms; do not allow the shoulders to hunch up to your ears. • Ensure that the ball is resting on the pelvis, not on the rib cage.

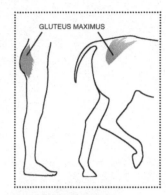

gluteals in man and beast

The human is one of the few mammals and the only primate to walk completely upright. Because of this, as compared to chimps, dogs, or horses we have the biggest gluteal muscles. Gluteus maximus is the big meaty muscle of the buttock; in humans it is one of the strongest in the body. It is a major hip extensor and it rotates the leg outward. Gluteals stabilize the pelvis when walking or moving the legs and they work hard in running or walking up a hill.

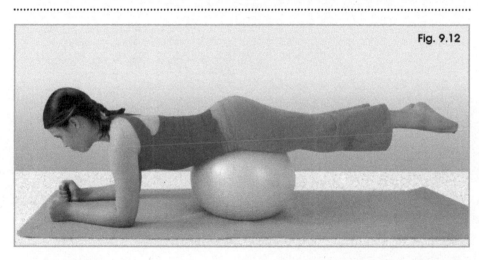

Fig. 9.12

starting position

Kneel with the ball in front of you. Walk out on your hands and place the elbows down on the mat; make your hands into fists, palms facing inward. Keeping your shoulders down, lean on the elbows. Your pelvis should be resting on the ball **(fig. 9.12)**.

movement 1: on elbows

1. Once you have correctly placed your elbows and hands on the mat, extend

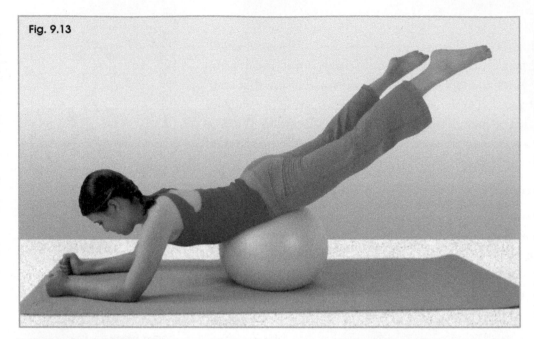

Fig. 9.13

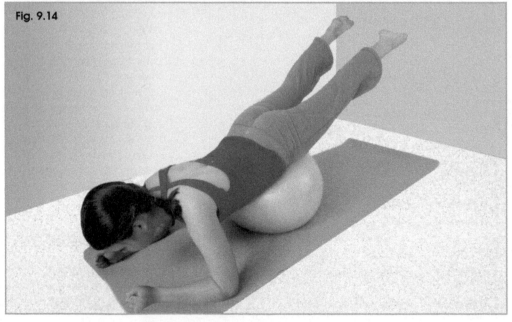

Fig. 9.14

your legs behind you **(fig. 9.13)**. Keep your navel pulled in toward your spine and hold the position for 2 or 3 breaths.

2. Come out of this dynamic position by walking the hands back toward the ball. Hang over the ball and rest.

movement 2: open and close legs

1. Placing your elbows again on the mat, take the starting position.

2. Open the legs evenly to shoulder-distance apart **(fig. 9.14)**. Pause for one breath.

3. Now squeeze the legs together.

4. Repeat four to six times, then walk the hands back toward the ball and hang over it.

Side Star

This is a fun exercise that will test your balance. Try to coordinate the foot and arm movements and keep the hips squared to the front. The other hand could be down on the mat for support. Test your balance by lifting the hand off the ground and onto the ball. The way the supporting foot is placed on the mat is essential to the success of this move. Angle the foot and "grind" it into th mat. The arm and leg work simultaneously: as the leg lifts so does the arm. Make sure the area around you is cleared of furniture.

Purpose To strengthen the core and practice balance.

Watchpoints • Keep your core very stable and straight. • Do not allow your shoulders to lift.

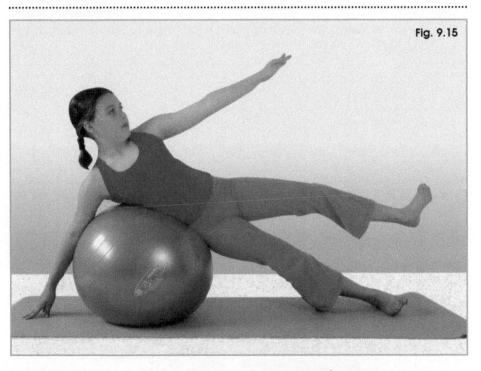

Fig. 9.15

starting position

Kneel beside the ball and shift the side of your rib cage onto the ball. Your fingertips could dangle down on the mat for support. Stretch one leg out to the side and dig the side of the foot into the mat.

movement: the star

1. Find your balance and slowly lift the upper leg, keeping it straight as you flex the foot. The arm lifts at the same time **(fig. 9.15)**.
2. Repeat three or four times.
3. Change sides and repeat.

Throw and Catch

I love this exercise because it is a fun and terrific workout for the lower body but also for the hands. The hands play multitudinous and important roles in our lives; they are also shock absorbers. Like adults, young people use their hands all day to grasp, push, pull, and manipulate objects, as well as to break falls and catch things. Keeping the small muscles of the hands well trained can help a person avoid injuries in sports activities. Throw and Catch gives your hands the attention they deserve while training coordination and building strength in the arms, legs, and hips.

Purpose To build strength in the abdominals, legs, and hips, and to train hand-to-eye coordination. To learn to properly use the hands while catching.

Watchpoints • Make sure the area around you is free of furniture and breakable objects. • Make sure the elbows are slightly bent to absorb shock as you catch the ball.

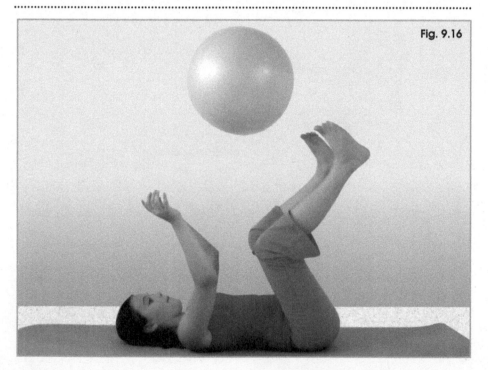

Fig. 9.16

starting position

Lie on your back with the ball between your ankles.

movement 1: feet to hands

1. Bend your knees and fling the ball up into the air **(fig. 9.16)** and catch it with your hands.

2. Repeat six to eight times.

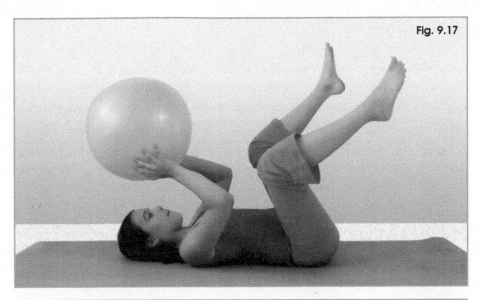

Fig. 9.17

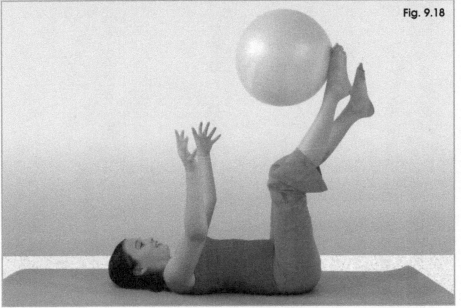

Fig. 9.18

movement 2: hands to hands

1. Lie on your back with the ball between your hands **(fig. 9.17)**.
2. Bend your elbows and toss the ball in the air, catching it between your hands.
3. Repeat six to eight times.

movement 3: hands to feet

1. Lie on your back with the ball between your hands.
2. Bend your elbows and toss the ball in the air, bouncing the ball off your toes or the front of your foot **(fig. 9.18)** and catching it with your hands.
3. Repeat six to eight times.

Ball Squat for Two

Coordination and cooperation is necessary to keep the ball level and to maintain balance as you work with your partner. Keep the spine in neutral, meaning let your tailbone drop down between your pelvis and not curl around the ball. Ensure that the center of the kneecap tracks over the second toe as you squat.

Purpose To strengthen the legs and feet and develop coordination and balance.

Watchpoints • Don't bend the knees too deeply—the heels should not come off the floor.

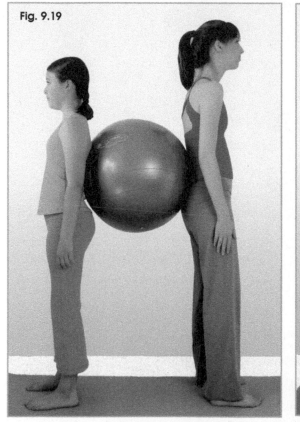

Fig. 9.19

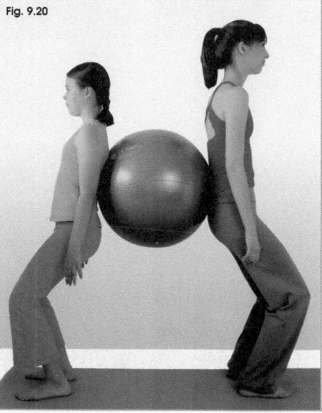

Fig. 9.20

starting position

Stand back to back with the ball between your lower backs. The feet are shoulder-distance apart and parallel **(fig. 9.19)**.

movement: parallel squat

1. Keeping both bodies upright, slowly bend the knees **(fig. 9.20)**.
2. Hold for a few seconds at the bottom of the movement and then slowly return to the starting position.
3. Repeat five to eight times.

Teaser for Two

Here is a challenge for the abdominals and a fun exercise to do with a partner. Work at your own pace, coming up as high as you can. You will try and roll through the spine one bone at time as you peel the body off the mat to go up into the air, aiming your fingertips, or in this case the small ball, toward your partner's shoulders.

Purpose To tone the abdominals.

Watchpoints • Make sure your partner is not too close to you. • Lift from the chest as you peel up. • Your feet should not move at all on your partner's thighs.

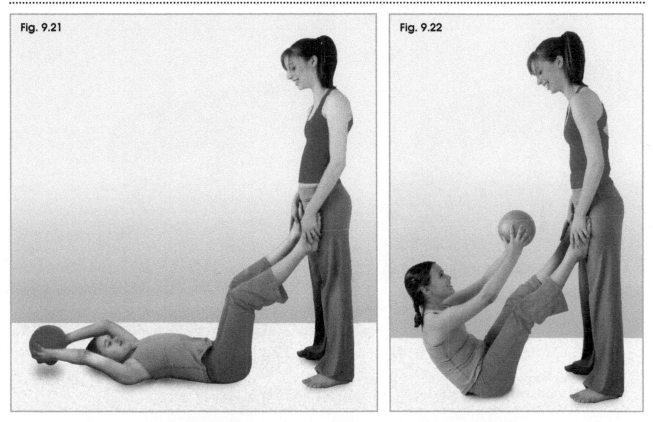

Fig. 9.21   Fig. 9.22

starting position

Lie on the mat. Keeping your knees bent, place the soles of your feet on your partner's thighs. Holding a small ball, take your hands overhead (fig. 9.21).

movement: the teaser

1. Raise your arms to the ceiling and slowly peel up off the mat, reaching your fingertips in the direction of your partner's shoulders. When you have come up as high as you can, pause (fig. 9.22).
2. Return the body slowly to the mat.
3. Repeat three to five times and change partners.

Balance Test

All the muscles in the core work to ensure balance. Begin by cautiously placing your knees on the ball and just lift the toes an inch or two. From there, graduate to balancing on your hands and knees. Make sure the space around you is completely clear of objects in case you lose balance. You may want to have someone spot you at first, or you may want to use the more stable Physio Roll (shown here).

Purpose To challenge core and balance.

Watchpoints • Master one step before you move to the next. • Work in a large empty space.

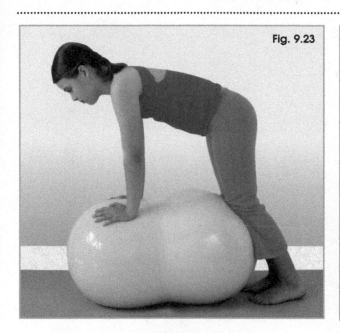

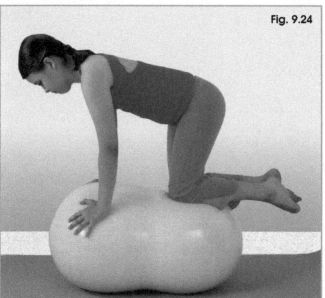

starting position

Stand behind the ball and place your hands shoulder-distance apart on the ball **(fig. 9.23)**.

movement: on the hands and knees

1. Taking your time, slowly shift your weight onto the ball so that only your toes are dangling on the mat. The knees are slightly apart.
2. When you're ready, lift your toes from the mat and hold in the kneeling position for as long as possible **(fig. 9.24)**.
3. Repeat three to five times.

Balls can form a bridge between the generations. Just as all ages can get together to kick a ball around before a family dinner, so a family can make room for partner activities and weight training on the ball. In the next chapter are exercises that can be enjoyed not only by older adults but by the entire family.

Check In: Solutions for Inactive Families

Computer games, surfing the web, and chatting online all take their tolls on young growing bodies by causing headaches and neck aches in the short-term and postural problems and eye strain in the long-term. Play is an important component to the healthy physical and mental development of children and ball playing develops the sensorimotor system, eye-hand coordination, and proprioception. In addition to ballwork, parents and schools must begin to improve students' health now by adding bone-stressing activities like jumping, skipping, and hopscotch into everyday life.

If you are worried about the health and activity level of your family, take heart. You have the power to create a nurturing home environment where real change can occur.

Do

- Be a role model and initiate activities that can be done as a family: gardening, walking, hiking, cycling, swimming, skiing, skating, or dancing.
- Encourage kids to play outdoors even if this involves hiring a physically active babysitter who will keep them moving.
- Focus on health, not weight, and compliment your teenagers on their accomplishments instead of focusing on appearances. Check out the website www.familyfitnessmatters.com for innovative weight-management programs for children and their families and the Canadian Association for Advancement of Women and Sport and Physical Activity (www.caaws.com) for programs and resources to encourage girls and women to be active.
- Promote an appreciation of all sizes and shapes by eliminating negative comments about people in the streets or on TV.
- Ensure that computer desks at home and at school are adjusted for your child's size. Stations for laptops need to be different than for desktop computers. Promote proper posture and frequent breaks.
- Pressure school boards to encourage children to spend more class time

in physical education and other activity classes. Put pressure on the big food companies and fast-food chains, but know that the real change in terms of diet must begin at home, where children should be educated from a young age to avoid sugar-laden soft drinks and snacks.

Don't

- Limit food intake or focus on the amount of food a child eats. Instead, experts recommend educating kids about nutritional foods versus unhealthy choices.
- Focus on a child's weight or her dress size.
- Send negative body images about your daughter's or son's body. Experts agree that mothers, and fathers, need to realize that the messages they convey during adolesence and in the teen years resonate throughout a person's life.

10
Strength Training for Older Adults

A Tolstoyan Story

On a quiet, nondescript Moscow street is the winter home of the famous Russian writer Leo Tolstoy. Every day of the week except Mondays you can cover your shoes with sloppy slippers and navigate the wide staircase of this house-museum while recorded piano music filters through the empty rooms. The day I stepped into Tolstoy's upstairs drawing room, I felt I was discovering the eighteenth-century townhouse for myself. There were no ropes and tourist queues, only the elderly ladies stationed in each room who sat on guard. I leaned over the bowls of violets on the window ledge and imagined Tolstoy's wife, Sonya, moving around the room while the Russian pianist Rachmaninoff played the grand piano.

What else do I remember? I kept circling back to Tolstoy's study to survey the two solid barbells: large black balls at the ends of iron bars, positioned directly outside his study. Did Tolstoy pump iron each morning before sitting down at his sawn-off desk to complete the fate of Anna Karenina? Did he perform a series of bicep curls each time he escaped to this study from his wife's parties or the demands of a large family?

We know from Tolstoy's diaries and his biographers that in his last years he immensely enjoyed physical activity. In his late fifties he thought nothing of walking from Moscow to his summer home at Yasnaya Polyana, a distance of

130 miles. According to biographer Ernest J. Simmons, Tolstoy thoroughly relished these excursions, which took him five days; these walks would be the "best remembrances" of his life. Up into his seventies he also enjoyed physically toiling in the fields near his summer home.

On the day I visited Tolstoy's final Moscow dwelling and surveyed his old-fashioned barbells, I was coming directly from a visit with Liuda. I wrote about Liuda in the introduction to this book—she's the Russian woman in her early sixties who broke her hip on the day before New Year's Eve and was housebound for months.

The exercise sessions with Liuda had not been easy. Despite the fact that muscle begins to atrophy in as little as five days following immobilization, it was five months before the surgeon visited her and gave the all-clear sign to exercise. Because she could not get to a pool, to a rehabilitation center, or even out of her apartment, I felt intense pressure that the exercises we did together would make or break her recovery. Moreover, we only had three weeks together, three meetings a week, to set up a program: we needed to develop something simple enough for Liuda to be able to keep to long after I was gone.

Unlike Tolstoy, Liuda had no tradition of "taking exercise." Neither had she, I believe, ever lifted a weight before in her life. She had grown up in Soviet times; there was little culture for women of her age to meet in gyms or stroll in malls. What this meant was that I had to be totally flexible, alter the exercises often, and simplify the breathing patterns; I encouraged Liuda simply to breathe naturally as she performed the exercises. The whole process humbled me as a Pilates instructor, yet the truth is that Liuda's situation is typical of many people. As a personal trainer it's easy to forget that the world is made up of many different types of people, and most of them don't have barbells outside their studies.

After three weeks Liuda did claim to feel the benefits of her strength exercises. As with many beginners or nonexercisers, Liuda had a lot to gain. The weights and resistance-band exercises helped her start feeling strong in her upper body almost from the beginning, and her weakened hip and leg muscles had nowhere to go but toward improvement. Her energy had increased, she told me, and she was sleeping better. Most important of all: she began to enjoy the exercises and appeared to be doing them on her own between our sessions.

People today are living longer than they did in Tolstoy's day; the older adult population worldwide is expected to double by 2030. Many aging baby boomers, even those without serious injuries to motivate them, are beginning to wake up to the fact that they must prepare their bodies now to ensure independence and quality of life in a prolonged old age. Part of the preparation for a successful aging process is not only physical but emotional.

The Self-Fulfilling Prophecy of Aging

Our attitudes toward aging can be critical to how each and every one of us approaches the aging process. Researchers have found that optimistic people live 7.5 years longer than those who are depressed, anxious, and pessimistic. Even taking into account race, sex, and socioeconomic status, Dr. Becca Levy, a social psychologist at Yale, concluded that the attitude that people had toward their own aging was highly correlated with a long life.

Thomas Hanna also writes about the potent effects of expectation on aging. Hanna believes that the mental attitude people have about the aging process may cause things to turn out exactly as they expect. To expect the worst sets the body up to reinforce discomfort as a permanent condition, which then makes the body become resistant to improvement and self-healing. Hanna writes urgently of the need for "a pride of age," as how we interpret certain discomforts is crucial to how they will play out in our bodies.

Dr. Elaine Dembe, a Toronto chiropractor and author of *Passionate Longevity*, sent out an SOS to find "stand-out seniors." She listened to their

The human body—like the tires on a car, or the rug on a floor—wears longest when it wears evenly.
—Hans Selye

Strength Training, Balance, and Older Adults

The over-sixty-five group is the fastest growing age group in our society. According to exercise physiologist Douglas S. Brooks, the most important thing older adults can do for themselves is strength training. He notes the important aspects of cardiovasular endurance for all ages but attests that the effects of strength training upon middle-aged and older populations is life changing. Miriam Nelson and other researchers at Tufts University have demonstrated that strength training can make older populations younger.

After strength training, the second most important training for older adults is in balance. Falls, and the fractures that follow, are the leading causes of death in people age seventy and older. Twenty percent of that age group who break a hip will die in the first year after the injury. Working with balls and other unstable surfaces helps older adults make the split-second adjustments necessary to avoid a fall. Strength training helps balance by keeping muscles strong and ready to react. Flexibility and agility training enhances the coordination necessary to maneuver through the environment safely.

heart health

Cardiovascular disease is the leading cause of death in men and women over age sixty-five. As we age the walls of the arteries can clog up with fatty substances that hamper the flow of blood to the heart and result in a heart attack. Men and women experience heart disease, heart attacks, and strokes differently. Learn the different symptoms—if you suspect that someone around you has these signs, get help immediately.

Healthy lifestyle choices such as a low fat diet, quitting smoking, and getting regular exercise will help prevent this killer disease. Aerobic exercises such as walking, swimming, and biking raise the heart rate, condition the heart muscle, and improve stamina. A well-conditioned heart does not need to work as hard to meet the body's demand for oxygen and it can pump more blood.

Exercise also contributes to the health of the capillaries and arteries—they dilate and circulate the blood easier.

inspiring stories and came up with ten secrets to passionate old age. The first secret highlighted the value of optimism: people who faced adversity and aging with hope and grace lived longer, more enjoyable lives. Other principles she discovered to be key to health and long life were tenacity, sociability, productivity, unity, mobility, vitality, responsibility, creativity, flexibility, and spirituality. Dr. Dembe reminds us that the secrets to living a longer, healthier life are within our reach and up to each of us to pursue.

It's strange to write a chapter on aging from a moment in my timeline when I am one year shy of my fiftieth birthday. Technically, I am middle-aged, but what do I really comprehend of aging in comparison with someone thirty years older than me?

Since the experts claim that inheritability is a significant factor in disease and the aging process, I look to my own parents for signs of how my aging might play out. I recall a time recently when I arrived in Arizona to visit them: they who had left their snowy home for a month to vacation. I stepped out of my back bedroom and paused in astonishment in front of my father—tanned and barefoot in his shorts and golf shirt—and my mom, down on her hands and knees on the rug figuring out a sewing pattern. My parents, almost thirty years older than me, were the pictures of youth.

Yet I can never forget for one moment that they are, like everyone else, caught in the inevitable flow of life. Each year the rules change a little more; I notice odd interactions popping up when I become the parent and they the children. As they age these interactions will continue until the parent role from their side is more and more muted. At seventy-four, my mother agreed to be shown in this book when I convinced her of how strongly I felt that older adults should be represented in a book on strength training. She may be an inspiration to aging women and men around the world, but I cannot forget that she is at the age when each year counts a lot. My father, seventy-seven, recently had a hip replacement and inspired us all by abandoning his walker four weeks after the operation in his determination to get back to walking, golf, and independence. Yet a new hip will never make him twenty again.

Who can put the brakes on the time wheel that affects us all, even my beloved three-legged tomcat, Monty? For a number of years I have been telling people that Monty is twelve (sixty-nine in human years) because I can't face his aging. Yet face it I must.

Youthful visions of age inspire us to remember that the golden years can be everything we want them to be. We have the opportunity to listen to each other in new ways. Our definitions of health and fitness expand to include relaxation, fun, spiritual pursuits, and healthy connections with friends and family. Or we hope they do. As yoga author Stephen Cope sagely writes: "All the yoga postures in the world cannot create the opening of the heart."

Older Adults and Exercise

"If I had known I'd live so long, I would have taken better care of myself" goes the old joke. Strength training may not shelter you from all the ravages of old age but it can provide a safeguard if illness strikes. "Skeletal muscle strength may not necessarily protect you against disease," claims Dr. Jeremy Walston, a gerontologist at Johns Hopkins. "But it can provide you with a reserve that can get you through the tough times" (*New York Times*, November 19, 2002).

If you haven't seen your doctor recently, undergo a medical exam before starting this or any exercise program. Many of the exercises in this book, not just the ones in this chapter, are suitable for older adults, but check first with your doctor. For older adults who cannot get down on the mat, many of the exercises can be done on a firm bed or a padded table.

The warm-up is especially important for older bodies. When the body is cold, muscles are more easily pulled and joints damaged. A proper warm-up increases the heart rate, increases the flow of blood through the tissues, and prepares the heart for action. Just as one warms the body for a game of golf by going through a couple of swings, before weight training start with a round of movement without weights. In addition, do some aerobic exercise like walking, or, if you are steady enough, bounce gently on a ball.

Take care how you bend over to lift free weights from the floor. Bend your knees and get close to the weights before you lift them; also take care when returning the weights to the ground. Keeping the weights on a rack or another surface besides the floor will also help in keeping the back healthy when lifting the weights in preparation for a workout.

When exercising with weights, keep your movements smooth and controlled—avoid jerky, ballistic movements. Also avoid rapid movements and quick twists or bending.

Monitor vital signs and stop if you feel any pain. Do not hold your breath; exercises should not interfere with normal breathing. If you do not feel secure enough sitting on a ball, use a Physio Roll or a chair to do the arm exercises.

Wear sneakers or rubber-soled shoes to avoid slipping. If you work out in a gym, review the safety tips on page 119.

Depending on your activity, a warm-down may be necessary, and it will certainly help reduce muscles aches. After vigorous walking or cycling, gradually slow down until your pulse is back to normal. Flexibility stretches are important at the end of your workout. Review stretching principles in chapter 7 and be sure to stretch after your workout, not before.

Sitting and Pelvic Movements

Sitting on the ball is active work and is therefore better for your posture and general back health than collapsing into a chair. If you are not stable on a ball, use a Physio Roll. To find neutral pelvis and optimal posture, do three bounces and then stop bouncing; your spinal curves should now be in proper balance. For movements 2 and 3, use the abdominal muscles to push and circle the ball.

Purpose To find optimal posture and learn mobility through the pelvis. Moving the pelvis from side to side and in circles loosens the low back.

Watchpoints • In movement 1, check in a mirror that you are sitting tall with the natural spinal curves in place. • Avoid overarching the back and popping out the rib cage. • Unassisted sitting is an endurance activity so don't overdo it. • Keep the chin horizontal, eyes level. In movements 2 and 3 do not force the movement. • Stop if you feel any pain.

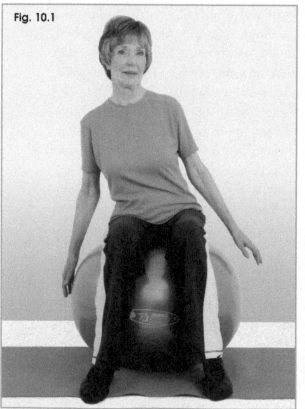

Fig. 10.1

starting position

Sit on the center of your ball, knees over ankles and your legs hip-distance apart. Your feet are parallel. If you feel unstable, widen the feet to shoulder distance. Pull the navel in toward the spine. Keep the chin level.

movement 1: sitting

1. Relax the shoulders.
2. As your fingertips relax toward the floor, let the weight of the body drop into the ball. Lengthen through the tips of the ears.
3. Sit for a number of minutes, breathing slowly and deeply. Add time as you get stronger.

movement 2: side to side

1. Keeping your feet firmly planted, use your abdominal muscles to shift your pelvis to the left, slightly lifting the left hipbone **(fig. 10.1)**. The ball will roll slightly.

2. Return to neutral pelvis.

3. Shift your pelvis to the right **(fig. 10.2)**.

4. Repeat six times to each side.

movement 3: full circles

1. Keeping your feet firmly planted, use your abdominal muscles to move the ball in a circle.

2. Draw five circles with your pelvis in one direction. Then reverse and circle your pelvis five times in the opposite direction.

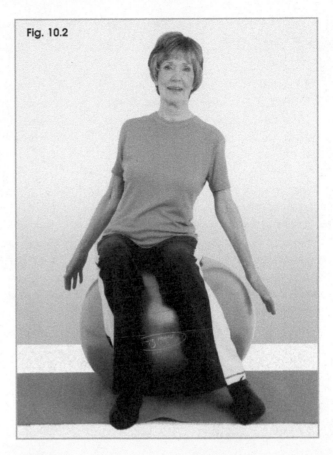

Fig. 10.2

Kegel Exercises and Incontinence

*O*ne of the many annoyances associated with getting older is incontinence. According to physiotherapist and urge incontinence expert Beate Carrière, stress or urge incontinence affects one in ten men, one in four women, and 17 percent of children between the ages of five and fifteen. Stress incontinence occurs when pressure within the abdomen causes urine to leak out involuntarily during coughing, laughing, or exertion. Kegels, invented by Dr. Arnold Kegel in the 1940s, are exercises that tone and strength the pubococcygius, the muscle that surrounds the opening of the vagina. More recently, exercise balls have been used by Carrière and others to rehabilitate patients with pelvic-floor dysfunction following pregnancy and other conditions. Specialized bouncing on balls and diaphragmatic breathing help men and women retrain weak pelvic-floor and sphincter muscles. A strong pelvic floor is as important for men as for women, because the pelvic floor muscles support the internal organs. A deficiency in these muscles can cause urinary problems at any age.

For more information on these exercises see Beate Carrière's video and book, *Exercises for the Pelvic Floor*, listed on the resources page.

213

How to Guard Someone on a Ball

Physical therapist and exercise ball pioneer Joanne Posner-Mayer explains that three or four gentle bounces will align the body correctly by putting the body's center of gravity over its base of support. Some people, however, do not feel secure enough to sit or bounce without support on a ball. Posner-Mayer suggests spotting a friend or a patient by kneeling in front of the person with your hands on her hips. The person being spotted should put her hands on the spotter's shoulders (fig. 10.3). If secure, she could bounce gently, perhaps swinging the arms. When your partner feels secure, the spotter moves back and guards her at the knees (fig. 10.4).

To help someone lie back on the ball, first have her sit tall. Guard her as she walks the feet slowly away from the ball (fig. 10.5). Continue to spot her as she continues to walk her feet out until the head is safely supported on the ball and the hips are lifted (fig. 10.6). To return to sitting, ask your partner to first place her hands behind her head and lift chin to chest. Then she should retrace her steps back toward the ball as she places her hands on the ball. Guard her until she is safely sitting upright on the ball, for this maneuver looks easier than it really is.

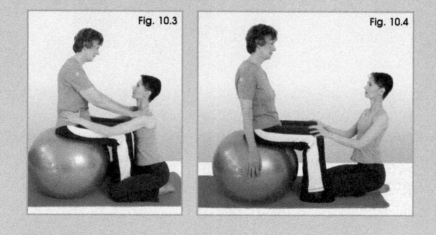

Fig. 10.3

Fig. 10.4

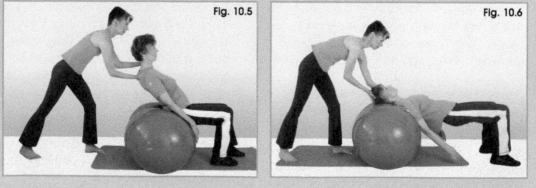

Fig. 10.5

Fig. 10.6

Resistance-Band Arm Work

Sitting on the ball while you perform the arm work is especially helpful for those with tightness in the hips, hamstrings, and low back. Keep the back in neutral—neither totally flattened nor in an exaggerated curve—and engage the abdominals. Try to keep your shoulder blades sliding down your back without forcing them down or squeezing them together. For added challenge place one foot on a small soggy ball. The unstable surface calls forth greater neuromuscular control and balance, but if you feel your posture is being compromised return both feet to the ground. In movements 3, 4, and 5 we set up the exercise with the resistance coming from the back. Place the band widely across the midback and shoulders and under the armpits. Begin with a taut band for all movements.

Purpose Movement 1 strengthens the shoulder abductor muscles; movement 2 strengthens the shoulder flexors; movement 3 strengthens the triceps and shoulder blade stabilizers. The abdominals and spine extensors work to stabilize the body.

Watchpoints • Avoid jerky movements and try not to use momentum to help you. • Take care that elbows do not lock or hyperextend. • Gently draw the navel in toward the spine.

starting position

Sit on the center of your ball, knees over ankles, legs hip-distance apart, feet parallel. Pull the navel toward the spine. Keep the chin level.

movement 1: shoulder abduction

1. Hold the band shoulder-width apart, resting your hands on your knees. Sit tall.
2. On the exhalation, keeping the elbow straight, slowly raise the right arm to the side **(fig. 10.7)**. The left arm remains on the knee.

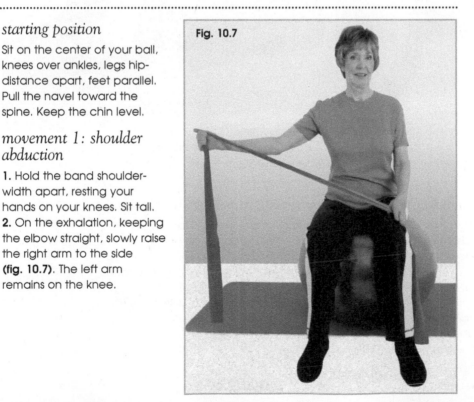
Fig. 10.7

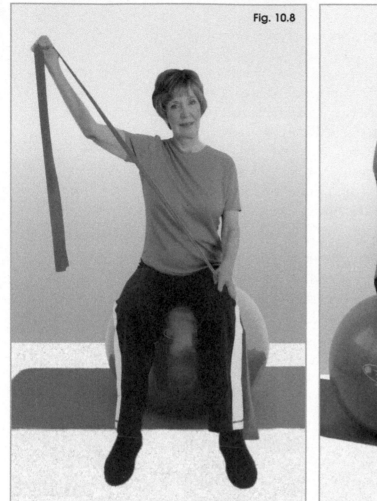

Fig. 10.8

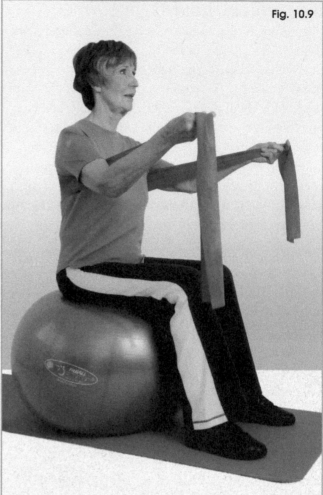

Fig. 10.9

3. Inhale to return to the starting position.
4. Repeat eight to ten times and change arms.

movement 2: shoulder flexion

1. Hold the band shoulder-width apart, resting your hands on your knees. Point the right thumb toward the ceiling. Inhale.
2. On the exhalation, keeping the elbow straight and the left hand on the knee, slowly raise the right hand upward until the arm is well above the shoulder **(fig. 10.8)**.

3. Inhale to return to the starting position. The band should remain taut.
4. Repeat eight to ten times and then change arms.

movement 3: pulling straight out

1. Wrap the band widely across the back of the rib cage and under the armpits. Inhale to prepare.
2. Exhale to straighten the arms out at shoulder height **(fig. 10.9)**.
3. Inhale to bend the arms, keeping the band taut. Exhale to straighten the arms.
4. Repeat six to eight times.

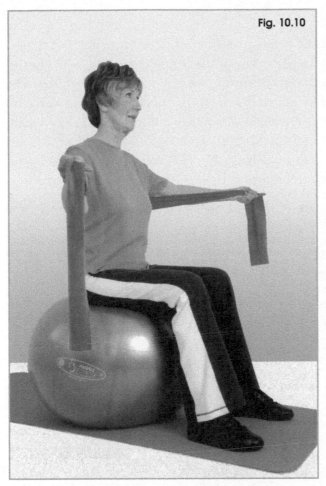

Fig. 10.10

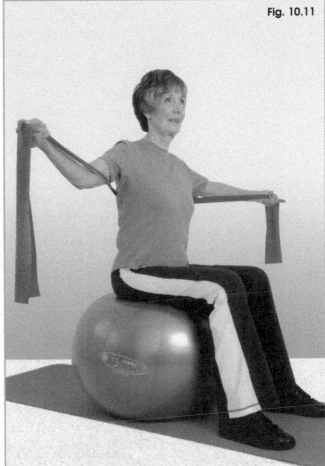

Fig. 10.11

movement 4: pulling out at 45 degrees

1. Start with the band taut and the elbows pointing into the waist.
2. Exhale to stretch the arms out on a 45-degree angle **(fig. 10.10)**.
3. Inhale to return.
4. Repeat six to eight times.

movement 5: pulling out at 90 degrees

1. Reach your arms directly out to the side. The palms are facing slightly forward. Inhale.
2. Exhale to stretch the arms out to a 90-degree angle **(fig. 10.11)**.
3. Inhale to return.
4. Repeat six to eight times.

Bridges

The Bridge, like the Plank, is a fundamental exercise for people of all ages. Both exercises require stabilization of the trunk and core. The Bridge strengthens the back of the legs, including the buttocks and hamstrings. The abdominals work to create a long line from the shoulders through the hips, knees, and ankles. Don't overextend the spine by lifting the pelvis too high. Holding the Bridge for a few seconds works endurance into the muscles. Keep the exercise small if you have low-back pain. To challenge yourself in movement 3, take away the base of support.

Purpose To work the back of the legs, hamstrings, buttocks, and the deep abdominal core.

Watchpoints • Do not overarch at the top by lifting the pelvis too high. • Be sure your neck is relaxed.

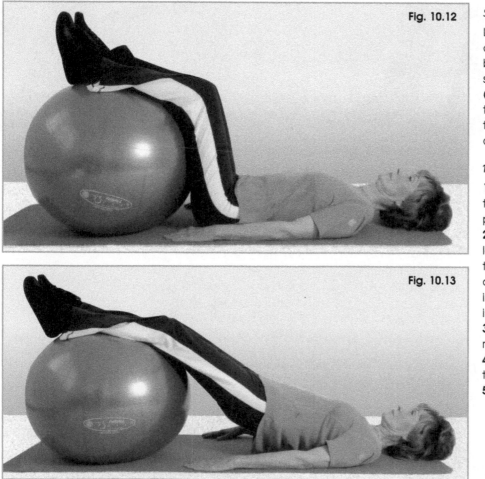

Fig. 10.12

Fig. 10.13

starting position

Lie on your back with your calf muscles resting on the ball and your hands by the side of your thighs **(fig. 10.12)**. Connect through the inner thighs so that your legs don't splay open.

movement 1: bridge

1. Inhale to lengthen the tailbone away from the pelvis.
2. Exhale to continue to lengthen and reach the tailbone up one vertebra at a time until your body is in a straight line, shoulders in line with toes **(fig. 10.13)**.
3. Inhale at the top of the movement.
4. Exhale to slowly lower the pelvis to the mat.
5. Repeat six times.

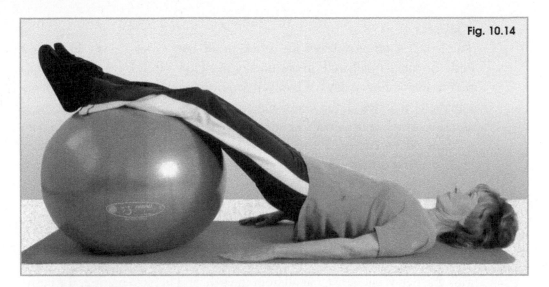

Fig. 10.14

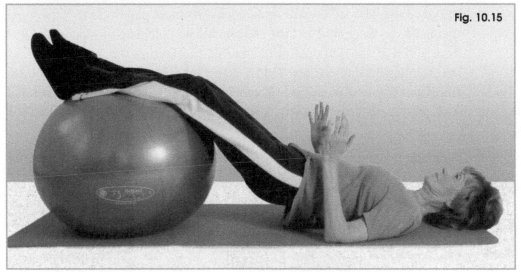

Fig. 10.15

movement 2: hold

1. Inhale to lengthen the tailbone away from the pelvis.

2. Exhale to continue to lengthen and reach the tailbone up one vertebra at a time until your body is in a straight line, shoulders in line with toes.

3. Stay here, breathing naturally, and hold for a few counts **(fig. 10.14)**.

4. Slowly return the pelvis to the mat. Repeat.

movement 3: take away the base of support (intermediate)

1. Practice the same movement as above, except this time lift your forearms off the mat when your pelvis is up **(fig. 10.15)**.

2. Breathing naturally, hold for a few counts.

3. Slowly return the pelvis to the mat. Repeat.

Planks

The ball is a wonderful tool for people of all ages to master the Plank and push-up. Since it only rolls in one direction, a Physio Roll gives you more support than an ordinary ball. When performing a push-up it's not only the large superficial muscles of the chest and triceps that are working. The serratus anterior, which runs under the armpit to attach to the ribs, and the middle sections of the trapezius, a muscle running from the spine to the shoulder blade, work together to keep the scapula in the proper position. When force is exerted as it is in a push-up and the shoulder blades are not in their proper tight-against-the-rib-cage position, injury can occur because unstable shoulder blades do not create a proper base from which to move or stabilize the arms.

Keep the movement very small when you're learning. You do not have to walk the hands out very far at all from the ball, and in movement 2, the push-up, you don't need to bend the arms much—it's more important that the spine and head stay in neutral and the abdominals are pulled up to support the low back and that you don't sag in the midriff. Ensure that the legs are together and the buttock muscles are slightly activated. The shoulder area is also an important part of this exercise. Watch for shoulder blades that "wing" out and look prominent. Ideally we try to keep the shoulder blades tight against the rib cage.

Purpose To strengthen the triceps, pectoral muscles, serratus, and other shoulder stabilizers and the inner core and to practice balance.

Watchpoints • Keep shoulder blades down, not lifted up by the ears. • The elbows are slightly soft, not locked or hyperextended. • Don't let the head drop: keep it in line with the spine.

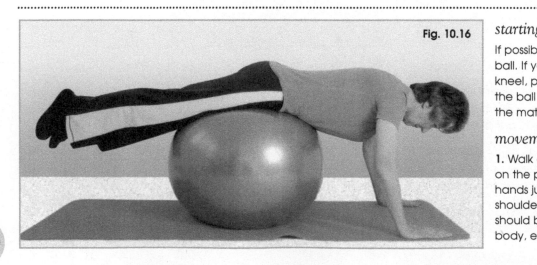

Fig. 10.16

starting position

If possible, kneel facing the ball. If you cannot safely kneel, place your body on the ball and your hands on the mat.

movement 1: plank

1. Walk out until the ball is on the pelvis, keeping the hands just wider than the shoulders. The fingertips should be parallel to the body, elbows slightly

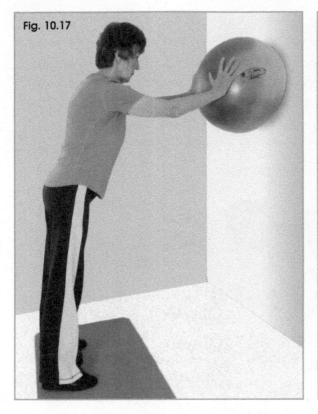

Fig. 10.17

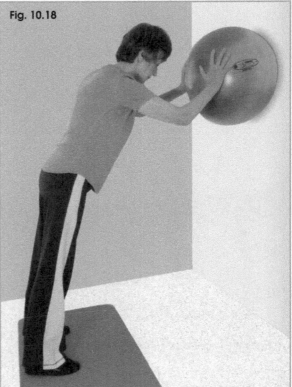

Fig. 10.18

angled back. Don't let the abdominal muscles drop.

2. Hold this position for a few seconds, breathing naturally **(fig. 10.16)**.

3. Return by walking the hands back in the direction of the ball.

4. To add challenge, walk out further so that the ball is on the thighs. Don't sag in the midriff.

movement 2: ball push-up on wall

1. Place the ball against the wall and your hands on the ball **(fig. 10.17)**.

2. Keeping the shoulders down, inhale to bend the elbows **(fig. 10.18)** and exhale to straighten them. Keep the abdominals engaged.

3. Repeat six to eight times.

Hamstring Curls with Two Balls

This is a challenging balance exercise that works the abdominals, arms, and wrists while strengthening the muscles of the buttocks and the back of the legs. Place the small, soft ball between the ankles before you walk out into the plank position. Hold the soft ball between the ankles as you bend and straighten your legs, trying to touch your heels to your buttocks. Straighten the legs back to the starting position with control, trying not to move the rest of the body. Keep your abdominals lifted up so that your low back does not sag.

Purpose To strengthen the hamstrings and calf muscles. Holding the extended position strengthens the abdominals, arms, and back muscles.

Watchpoints • Do not overarch the low back. • Keep the body straight in the plank position, navel lifted. • Distribute the weight evenly between both hands. • Don't allow the hips to drop. • Gaze down on the mat and don't let the head sag.

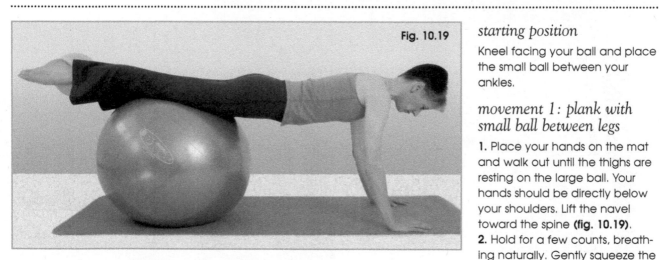

Fig. 10.19

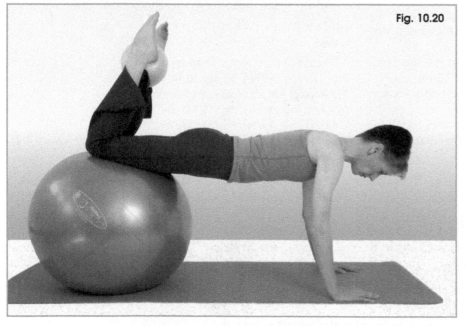

Fig. 10.20

starting position

Kneel facing your ball and place the small ball between your ankles.

movement 1: plank with small ball between legs

1. Place your hands on the mat and walk out until the thighs are resting on the large ball. Your hands should be directly below your shoulders. Lift the navel toward the spine **(fig. 10.19)**.

2. Hold for a few counts, breathing naturally. Gently squeeze the small ball.

3. Pick the hands up, walk back to the large ball, and relax over it.

movement 2: hamstring curl

1. Keep the small ball between the ankles. Place your hands on the mat and walk out until the thighs are resting on the large ball. Hands should be below the shoulders. Lift the navel toward the spine.

2. Breathing naturally, bend the knees to bring the ball slowly almost to the buttocks **(fig. 10.20)**. Pause, then slowly extend the legs.

3. Repeat six to eight times, then release the smaller ball and walk the hands back to the supporting ball. Relax over the supporting ball.

Hans Selye, the father of stress research, believes that an ever-increasing proportion of the human population dies from wear-and-tear diseases—degenerative conditions—that are primarily due to physical and emotional stress. Selye suggests that we voluntarily equalize the physical stress on our bodies by varying our activities in such a way that stress is shifted from one part of the body to the other. The check-in below will help you monitor your posture and give you some ideas on how to add variety to your strength workout.

Following the check-in are three thirty- to forty-minute, upper- and lower-body strength-training workouts: a restorative workout for those recovering from injuries or returning to exercise; a basic workout for those who have no limitations or injuries but are just beginning; and an intermediate workout for those who are fit and strong. Start with three sessions a week and try to complete one level before moving on to the next.

Check-In: Posture Control and How to Complement Your Strength Workout

It's good to monitor your posture throughout the day. Start by asking yourself if your shoulders are up by your ears. If so, why? Is there pain in the shoulder area? Are you anxious? Has this habit become so natural that you are only aware of it when you pause a few times during your day to notice your posture?

It's impossible for anyone to remain in good posture all day; use certain cues throughout your day to assess your body's bearing in any given moment. One trick is to wear an elastic band on the wrist. When you see it, think "sit up straight." When you enter the bathroom check your posture in the mirror. When you're walking, be aware of whether your head has dropped and your eyes are focused on the ground. Throughout the day when you see or feel the elastic on your wrist ask yourself: Are my shoulders rolling forward? Do I feel open across the collarbones?

Remember that the abdominals are essential to maintaining good posture. Draw the navel gently toward the spine rather than "sucking in" the belly, as this distorts the body.

Whether you're lifting a parcel from the ground or reaching overhead, learn to contract the abdominal core to protect the low back. Don't forget about the other deep postural muscles in the hip, back, shoulders, and abdominals. Work with a physical therapist or other postural specialist if necessary to make sure you are activating the correct muscles to make the low back safe. Get regular check-ups that include a postural assessment. Do balance exercises to test your core and your balance.

It's important to add aerobic activities to your strength workout. My three favorite activities are walking, swimming, and cycling.

Walking is versatile and can be used for transportation or relaxation and it is suitable for all sorts of fitness levels. Walking is low impact: it works the muscles of the legs without straining the joints. Walk outdoors or indoors on a treadmill but walk in good posture, keeping the shoulders relaxed and the head up. Keep your arms moving and tucked in close to the body. Sore ankles may be the result of improper shoes and/or a tendency to roll the ankles in or out when you walk. Choose correct footwear that provides support. Take time to stretch out after a walk.

The experts recommend steady walking not only for cardiovascular health but also in healing low-back pain. Fast-paced walking with swinging arms is easier on the low back than slow walking or the stop-and-start walking associated with strolling and window shopping. Join a walking group or set up your own program alternating between normal-paced walking and periods of faster and more intense strides.

Cycling and swimming strengthen the heart, improve stamina, and help protect from heart problems. Cycling has the added advantage of balance practice; cycle only in areas that are not full of traffic. Good technique is essential on a bike. Be sure the bike is sized to fit you, including making sure that the seat is at the correct height. The legs should be able to extend fully on a pedal stroke with just a slight bend at the knee. Keep your upper body relaxed. Always wear a helmet.

Swimming is a very effective aerobic exercise. It works on the health of your heart while toning and strengthening the body. Swim laps or join an aqua-fit class.

Final Words

In the introduction we discussed the outstanding significance of function when designing a strength-training program. Functional movement imitates real life and the varied movements of sports activities. Most of us have been brought up believing that large, bulky muscles equate with a fit body, yet there are limitations to isolating specific muscle groups and building up some muscles at the expense of others.

A Pilates approach to optimal strength and balance works the body from the inside out. The small muscles of the body are designed to provide support for the spine: its joints, discs, and ligaments. When the spine is stable and the abdomen is strong, the hips, knees, and shoulders can work efficiently and safely.

Research attests that it is never too late or too early to begin a strength-training program: ten years is ideal. Attitude and openness is essential when approaching a new method—perhaps more important than any physical advantages you may bring to the gym or Pilates class. Being open is not only about being willing to try new things. It also means reconsidering what you already know. Even if you have had some experience with balls and unstable surfaces, a Pilates approach may feel very different from what you are used to. Perhaps you are well versed in Pilates; yet the first time you work out with a ball may challenge and surprise you. Pay attention: the ball can bring out the show-off in some people, the scaredy-cat in others. Use common sense and listen to your own body.

Working the body from the inside out is not about going through the motions. It's about infusing meaning into each movement, no matter how small. In *The Pilates Method of Physical and Mental Conditioning*, one of the first books ever written about the Pilates Method, Philip Friedman and Gail Eisen wrote: "A few well-designed movements, properly performed in a balanced sequence, are worth hours of doing sloppy calisthenics or forced contortions." With Pilates you are using the mind to control the body and practice will help you master the moves. Many of you may enjoy the benefits almost at once; some students report feeling taller and stronger even after a couple of sessions. If you are beginning or returning to exercise after a long sedentary period, take heart. Remember the adage that you never forget how to ride a bike? The "computer" in your body has only to find the memory of this action and your body will re-create the move. Working out on a ball is unpredictable and unfamiliar, so be prepared to have your balance tested and improved upon.

My passion for the ball has given me the chance to teach workshops in many parts of the world. What has been wonderful about teaching workshops abroad is what I've had the opportunity to learn. With the help of knowledgeable translators (who were also often gifted physiotherapists) and the impressive level of expertise of the participants, I opened myself up in a way I might not have done back home. Working with other Pilates teachers, physiotherapists, and fitness professionals forced me to reevaluate my entire approach to weight training and to the Pilates exercises.

The Pilates Method, like many movement and bodywork fields, is constantly expanding as we learn more about the body and new research is adapted to different population groups, levels, and needs. The world of weight training is also going through its own evolution as more trainers and coaches use lighter weights, replace benches with unstable and mobile surfaces, work on one limb or a narrow base of support, and design programs that relate more closely to the functional movement demands of their athletes. With so much information and so many options available, it is important to greet new methods and trends with caution. But don't let caution stop you from continuing to learn, to try new things, to explore and grow.

Sometimes on the road, far from home, I find myself rereading favorite parts of Stephen Cope's *Yoga and the Quest for the True Self*, an eloquent book on the promise of yoga as spiritual and physical guide. Cope, influenced by thinkers such as Socrates, Carl Jung, and Jacob Needleman, has thought long and hard about successful teaching situations—transformational "cocoons" as he calls them, beneficial for both student and guide. Growth in any field means openness: to constantly circle back, revisit the work, and empty the mind of preconceived notions—especially your own preconceived notions.

Cope argues that in a truly effective teaching environment a "don't know mind" in both teacher and student is essential.

Ultimately, strength training is a solitary journey; a charismatic trainer can guide you, an inspiring book may provide a roadmap, yet only you can bring to this journey the perseverance and intelligence it deserves. Some impressions can be recorded in a journal, beside your number of repetitions and pounds lifted, yet many benefits cannot be seen. Pilates is not competitive so try not to compare yourself against others or against the spectre of your former self. Instead, keep in mind Stephen Cope's wise words: "The spiritual pilgrim needs three distinct qualities in approximately equal measure: common sense, skepticism, and openness."

Hopefully this book has given you many options and variations for approaching your strength-training sessions, whether you are working with the small therapeutic exercises with the more challenging moves. You should expect to find that your balance and posture will improve as the muscles that stabilize your spine, shoulders, hips, and knees begin to work more effectively, in ways for which they are designed.

Three strength-training workouts end this book. Restorative Strength Training is a gentle workout for those recovering from injuries or returning to exercise; Basic Strength Training is for those who are beginners to the ball and/or strength training but have no limitations or injuries; and Intermediate Strength Training, for those who are fit and strong and want to be challenged. Start with Restorative or Basic Strength Training and complete that level before moving up.

I suggest that you begin training with thirty- to forty-minute workouts three times a week, but remember that twice or even once a week is better than nothing. Fit the workouts into your life—and know that for some people this means literally writing each workout into your schedule.

Whatever level you choose, try to complete the entire workout, as each level is a complete workout in itself. Stick to the order the exercises are presented in; they are in order for a reason: to ensure you are warmed up before more vigorous moves and to facilitate a smooth transition onto or off of the ball. Stretches are put at the end of each workout so that you stretch when your muscles are warm.

Each strength workout has been laid out with thumbnail photos to provide a quick reference and to jog your memory of the exercise. The page numbers are supplied so that you can easily cross-reference back to the full instructions in the text. Work at your own pace and enjoy your workout.

WORKOUT 1:
Restorative
Strength Training

Workout 1: Restorative Strength Training

The goal of Restorative Strength Training is to locate and target some of the key stabilizers of the abdomen and low back. To do so we begin with some pre-Pilates exercises: miniscule movements that reprogram the body in a safe and functional way. Then to this new core strength and awareness we add larger moves, more resistance, and balance training. Work in good posture and alignment with a quality of movement that is controlled and precise. Eight or less repetitions per exercise is recommended. Remember to use the breath, especially the exhalation, to ensure that the deep core muscles of the low back and abdomen are fully engaged to protect the low back. *Gently* draw in your navel without sucking in your gut. Don't forget your pelvic floor, as these muscles connect through the nervous system to the deep abdominals. Think of an elevator lifting up and creating support for the entire abdominal area. If you have chronic pain it is essential that you check with your physical therapist or health care practitioner before you begin these exercises.

Navel-to-Spine (p. 38)

1. stabilizing on all fours

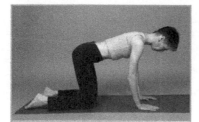

(avoid with knee problems)

Tailbone Curls (p. 40)

2. tilting the pelvis in and out of neutral

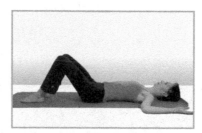

Heel Slides and Single-Leg Circles (p. 45)

3. heel slides

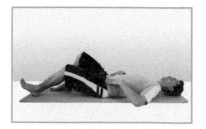

4. open knee

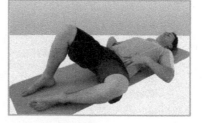

5. small single-leg circles

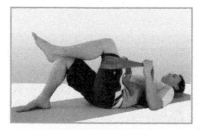

Scapula Isolation and Rib Cage Stability (p. 49)

6. scapula isolation

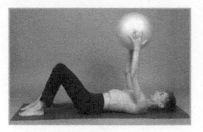

7. rib cage stability

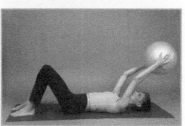

Ball Breathing (p. 22)

8. back breathing

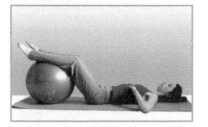

Chest Opener with Arm Circles (p. 24)

9. soldier arms on the mat

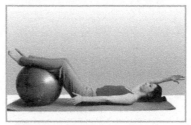

Pelvic Floor and Knee-Lift Stabilizing Exercise (p. 42)

10. locating the pelvic floor

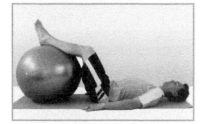

11. add hold

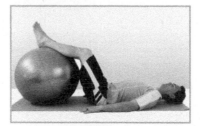

(hold for 3 to 5 seconds, breathing naturally)

12. feel the transversus abdominis

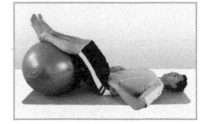

13. single-knee lift

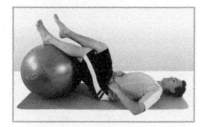

Abdominal Curls (p. 85)

14. ab curls, legs on the ball

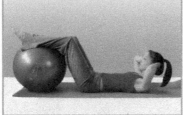

The Roll-up (p. 87)

15. half roll-up

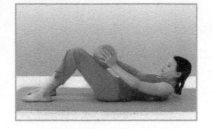

Heel Slides and Single-Leg Circles (p. 45)

16. single-leg circles on ball

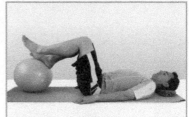

Single- and Double-Leg Stretches (p. 90)

17. single-leg stretch, modification

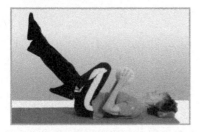

Extensions (p. 174)

18. navel-to-spine

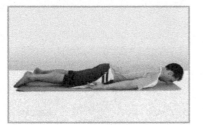

19. breaststroke preparation on mat

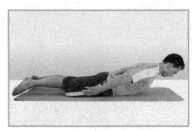

Balance Test 2: Standing (p. 74)

20. standing with closed eyes

21. single leg

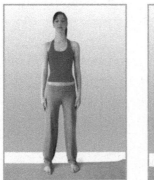
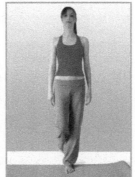

The Footwork Exercises (p. 62)

22. parallel feet

23. small turnout

24. calf raises

25. add weights

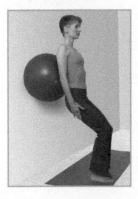 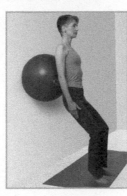 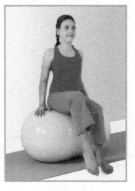 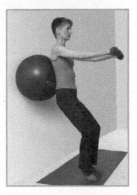

Planks (p. 220) *Balance Test 1: Sitting (p. 72)*

**26. ball push-up
on wall**

27. open eyes

28. lift foot

**29. narrow the base
of support**

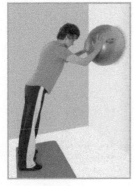 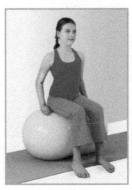 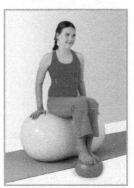 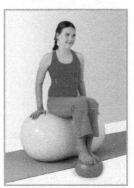

Sitting and Pelvic Movement (p. 212)

30. side to side

31. full circles

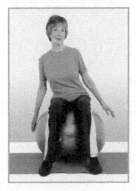 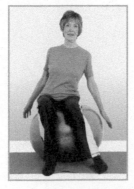

Sitting on the Ball: Upper Body (p. 168)

32. external rotation

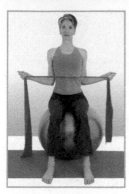

33. arm pull

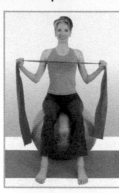

34. triceps

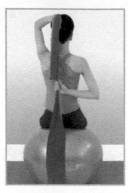

Resistance-Band Arm Work (p. 215)

35. shoulder abduction

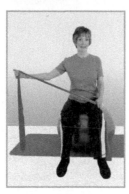

36. shoulder flexion

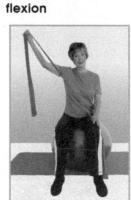

37. pulling straight out

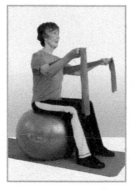

38. pulling out at 45 degrees

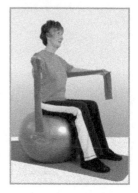

39. pulling out at 90 degrees

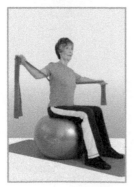

Half Roll-Downs with Resistance Band (p. 51)

40. half roll-down

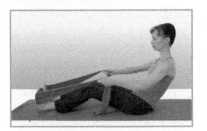

On the Mat: Lower Body (p. 171)

41. single-leg bend and stretch

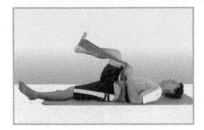

Single-Leg Stretch Series (p.145)

42. parallel leg

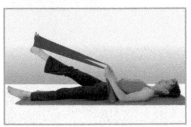

43. turnout

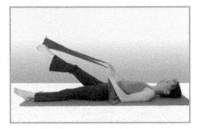

44. hamstring stretch

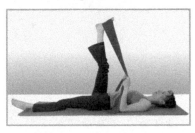

Bridges (p. 218)

45. bridge

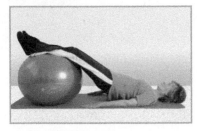

Inner Thigh Stretch (p.149)

46. frog stretch

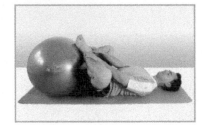

Hip Stretch (p. 150)

47. hip stretch

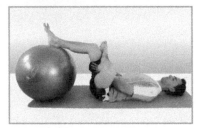

Spinal Twist (p. 151)

48. spinal twist

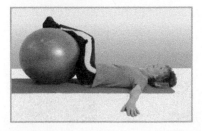

WORKOUT 2:
Basic Strength Training

Workout 2: Basic Strength Training

Make sure you can complete the Restorative level before moving up. You might be returning to exercises but you should have no injuries or limitations for this level. We begin with some breathing work and pre-Pilates exercises to make sure the deep core muscles are located and working. In your own time add more challenging moves.

Ball Breathing (p. 22)

1. side breathing

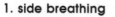

2. back breathing

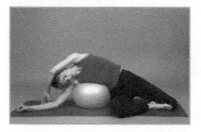

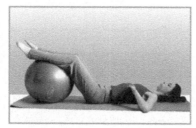

Chest Opener with Arm Circles (p. 24)

3. soldier arms on the mat

Breathing and The Hundred (p. 27)

4. the hundred (breath only)

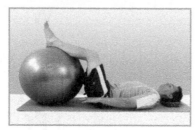

Pelvic Floor and Knee-Lift

5. locating the pelvic floor

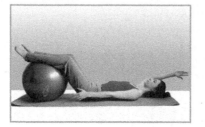

Stabilizing Exercise (p. 42)

6. feel the transversus abdominis

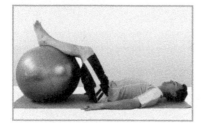

7. single-knee lift

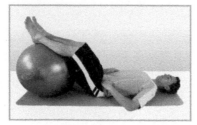

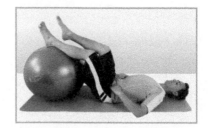

Abdominal Curls (p. 85)

8. ab curls, legs on the ball

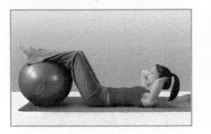

The Roll-up (p. 87)

9. half roll-up

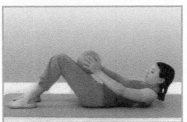

Single- and Double-Leg Stretches (p. 90)

10. single-leg stretch

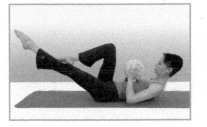

11. double-leg stretch

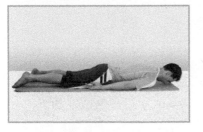

Extensions (p. 174)

12. navel-to-spine

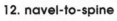

13. breaststroke preparation on mat

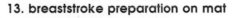

Oblique Twists (p. 93)

14. feet on the mat

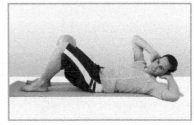

Knee-Lift Stablizing Exercise (p. 82)

15. knee-lift stabilizing exercise on small ball

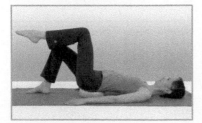

16. double-knee lift

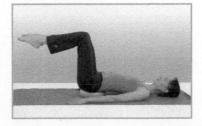

With the Small Ball (p. 95)

17. bicycle in air

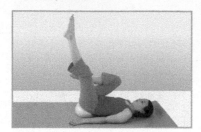

18. on the side, squeeze and lift

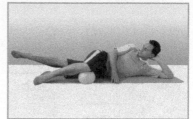

19. on the side, inner thighs

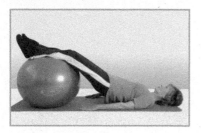

Bridges (p. 218)

20. bridge

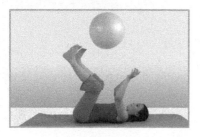

Throw and Catch (p. 200)

21. feet to hands

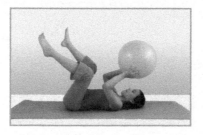

22. hands to hands

23. hands to feet

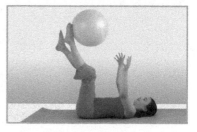

The Footwork Exercises (p. 62)

24. parallel feet

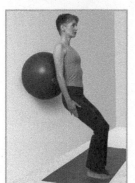

25. small turnout

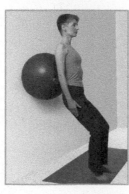

26. calf raises

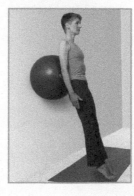

27. add weights

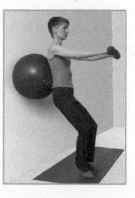

Balance Test 1: Sitting (p. 72)

28. lift foot

29. lift leg with rotation

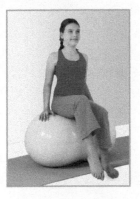 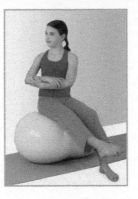

Sitting on the Ball:
Upper Body (p. 168)

30. external rotation

31. arm pull

32. triceps

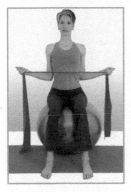 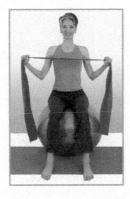 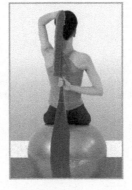

Resistance-Band Arm Work (p. 215)

33. shoulder abduction

34. shoulder flexion

35. pulling straight out

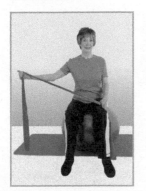 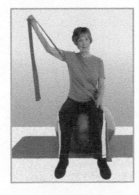 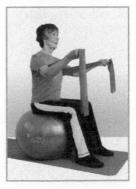

Resistance-Band Arm Work (p. 215) continued

36. pulling out at 45 degrees

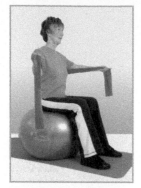

37. pulling out at 90 degrees

38. ab curls

Ab Curls on the Ball (p. 98)

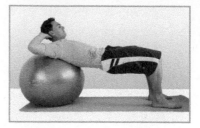

Ball as Bench (p. 112)

39. chest press

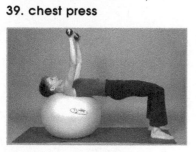

40. flies

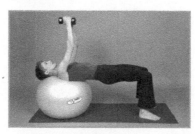

41. backstroke

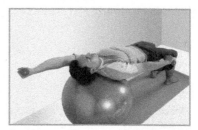

42. triceps isolator

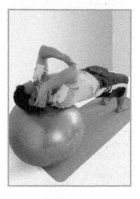

43. modification

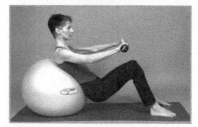

(use as starting position
if necessary)

On the Belly (p. 124)

44. single-arm row

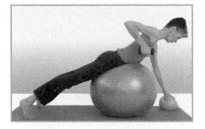

45. triceps targetter

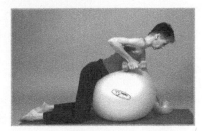

46. modification

(work on the knees if necessary)

Side-Lying Arm Work (p. 132)

47. shoulder rotation

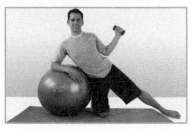

48. jab and extend

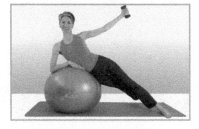

Bicep Curls / Wrist Curls (p. 129)

49. bicep curls on knees

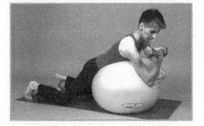

50. bicep curls on heels

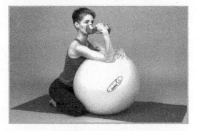

(start with small weights)

51. wrist curls: palms up

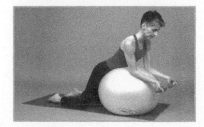

52. wrist curls: palms down

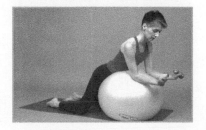

Extensions and Airplanes (p. 193)

53. the swan

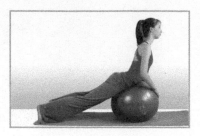

54. shell on the ball

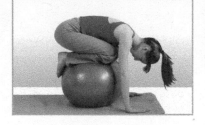

Planks (p. 220)

55. plank

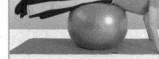
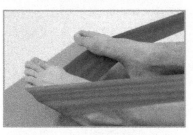

Roll Downs with Pull (p. 177)

56. roll down with pull

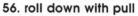
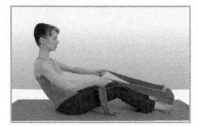

57. seated row

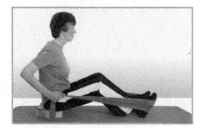

58. bend and stretch ankles

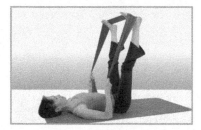

On the Mat: Lower Body (p. 171)

59. double-leg bend and stretch (parallel)

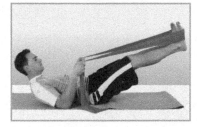

(head up or down)

60. double-leg bend and stretch (medial rotation)

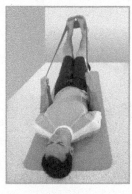

61. hip abduction

Single-Leg Stretch Series (p. 145)

62. hamstring stretch

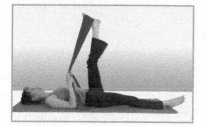

63. cross the midline

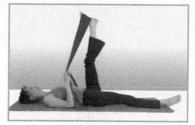

64. open the leg

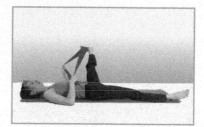

Hip-Flexor Stretch (p. 152)

65. basic

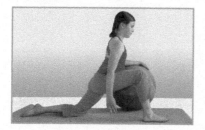

The Tabletop and Quad Stretch (p. 157)

66. the tabletop

67. with quad stretch

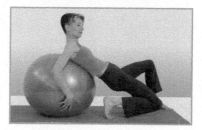

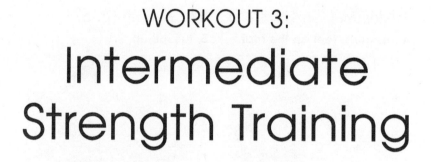

WORKOUT 3:
Intermediate Strength Training

Workout 3: Intermediate Strength Training

This workout is for those who are strong and who have mastered the basic workout and want to go further into the work. You could add more poundage to some of the weight exercises but remember that you are working in conjunction with a mobile surface. It is harder to stabilize your body on a ball than it is on a stable surface such as a machine, bench, or chair. Even though you may be adding more poundage, and more challenging moves, the goal is to gain strength without sacrificing precision or technique. To build endurance you should be moving smoothly from one move to the next without stopping.

Ball Breathing (p. 22)

1. back breathing

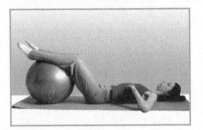

Breathing and The Hundred (p. 27)

2. breathing

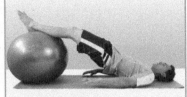

3. the hundred (breath only)

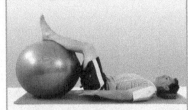

Abdominal Curls (p. 85)

4. ab curls, feet on the mat

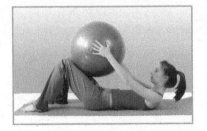

The Roll-up (p. 87)

5. full roll-up

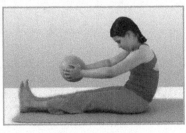

Single- and Double-Leg Stretches (p. 90)

6. single-leg stretch

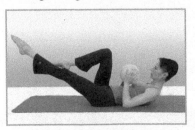

7. double-leg stretch

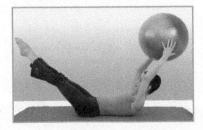

Extensions (p. 174)

8. breaststroke preparation on ball

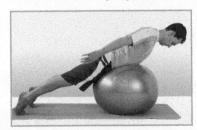

Oblique Twists (p. 93)

9. tabletop legs

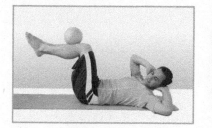

Knee-Lift Stablizing Exercise (p. 82)

10. knee-lift stabilizing exercise on small ball

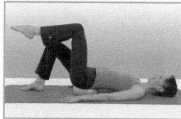

11. double-knee lift

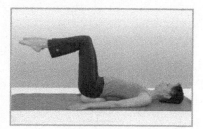

With the Small Ball (p. 95)

12. bicycle in air

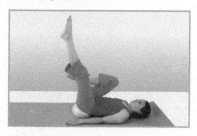

13. beats

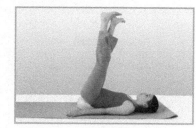

14. on the side, squeeze and lift

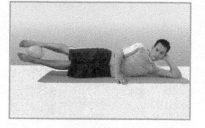

15. on the side, inner thighs

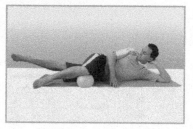

Inner Thigh Stretch (p. 149)

16. inner thigh stretch on small ball

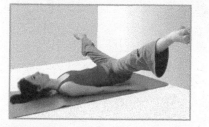

Bridges (p. 218)

17. take away the base of support

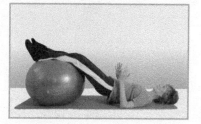

Abdominal Challenges (p. 100)

18. oblique challenge

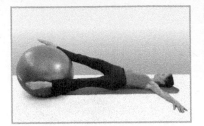

19. abdominal challenge

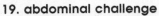
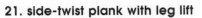

Side-Twist Plank with Leg Lift (p. 102)

20. side-twist plank

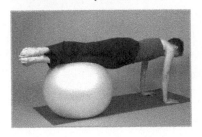

21. side-twist plank with leg lift

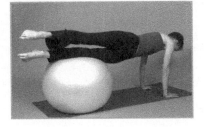

The Footwork Exercises (p. 62)

22. parallel feet

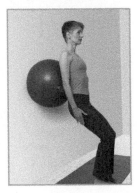

23. small turnout

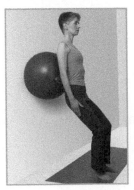

24. calf raises

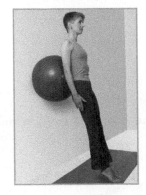

25. add weights

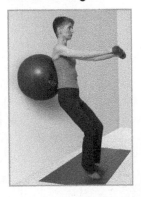

26. resistance band biceps curls

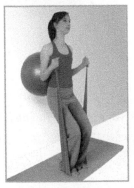

Squats with and without Weights (p. 67)

27. wide squat with biceps curls

28. side raises

29. isolate the belly of the muscle

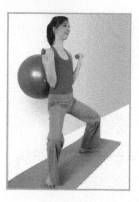

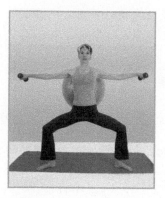

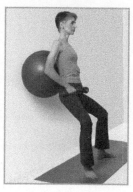

Single-Leg Footwork and Lunges (p. 69)

30. single-leg footwork, high half-toe

31. single-leg lunge

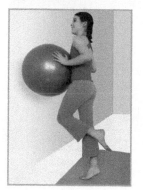

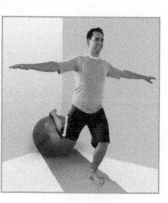

Sitting on the Ball with Weights (p. 134)

32. overhead press

33. side lift, small ball challenge

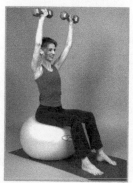

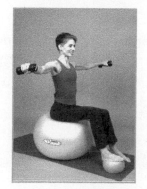

Ball as Bench (p. 112)

34. chest press

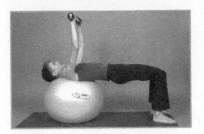

35. single-arm chest press with small ball

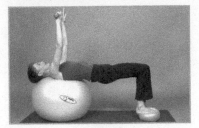

36. flies

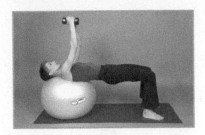

37. backstroke

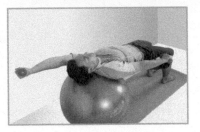

38. triceps isolator

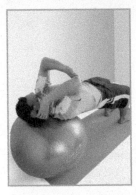

39. bicep curls on the back

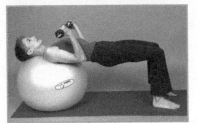

40. pullover with abdominal curl

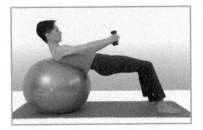

41. from side to side

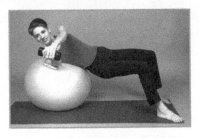

On the Belly (p. 124)

42. single-arm row

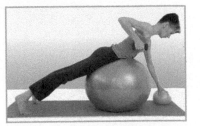

43. triceps targetter

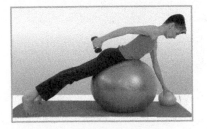

44. double-arm row

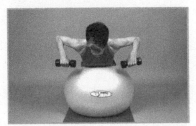

Side-Lying Arm Work (p. 132)

45. shoulder rotation

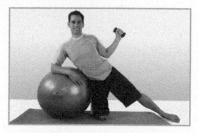

46. jab and extend

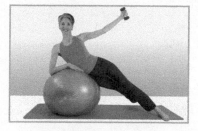

Bicep Curls / Wrist Curls (p. 129)

47. bicep curls on knees

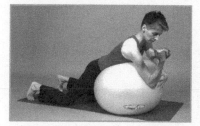

48. bicep curls on heels

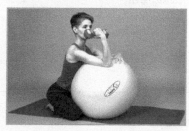

49. wrist curls: palms up

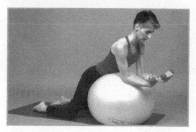

50. wrist curls: palms down

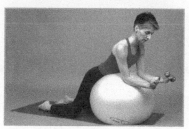

Extensions and Airplanes (p. 193)

51. the swan

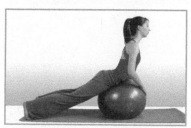

52. airplane

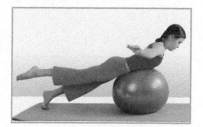

Extensions and Airplanes (p. 193) continued

53. shell on the ball

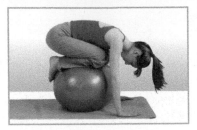

54. arabesque

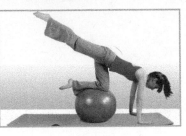

Hamstring Curls with Two Balls (p. 221)

55. plank with small ball between legs

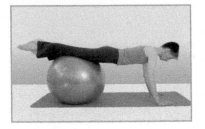

56. hamstring curl

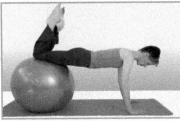

Side Star (p. 199)

57. the star

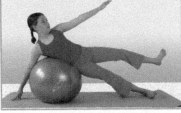

On Elbows (p. 197)

58. on elbows

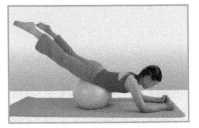

59. open and close legs

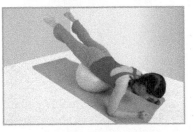

Balance Test (p. 204)

60. on the hands and knees

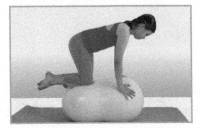

On the Mat: Lower Body (p. 171)

61. double-leg bend and stretch (parallel)

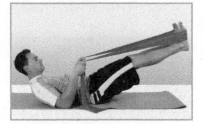

(head up or down)

62. double-leg bend and stretch (medial rotation)

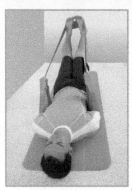

63. hip abduction

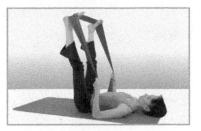

Single-Leg Stretch Series (p. 145)

64. hamstring stretch

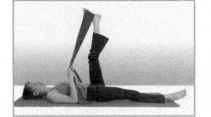

65. cross the midline

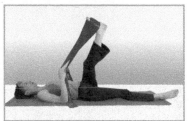

66. open the leg

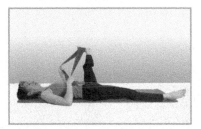

Hip-Flexor Stretch (p. 152)

67. intermediate

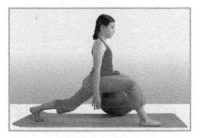

The Tabletop and Quad Stretch (p. 157)

68. the tabletop

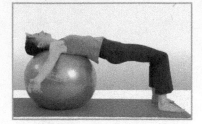

69. with quad stretch

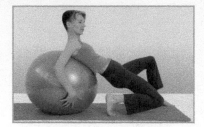

70. supported arch

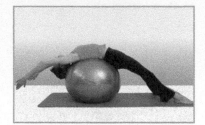

Resources

Books

Carrière, Beate. *The Swiss Ball: Theory, Basic Exercises and Clinical Application*. Germany: Springer-Verlag, 1998.

Cope, Stephen. *Yoga and the Quest for the True Self*. New York: Bantam Books, 1999.

Craig, Colleen. *Pilates on the Ball*. Rochester, Vt.: Healing Arts Press, 2001.

———. *Pilates on the Ball: A Comprehensive Book and DVD Workout*. Rochester, Vt.: Healing Arts Press, 2003.

———. *Abs on the Ball*. Rochester, Vt.: Healing Arts Press, 2003.

Dembe, Elaine. *Passionate Longevity*. Toronto: John Wiley & Sons Canada, Ltd., 2003.

Goldenberg, Lorne and Peter Twist. *Strength Ball Training*. Champaign, Ill.: Human Kinetics, 2002.

Hanna, Thomas. *Somatics*. Cambridge, Mass.: Perseus Books, 1988.

Hartmann, Thom. *The Edison Gene*. Rochester, Vt.: Park Street Press, 2003.

Jemmett, Rick. *Spinal Stabilization: The New Science of Back Pain (2nd ed.)* Halifax: Novont Health Publishing, 2003.

Jemmett, Rick. *The Athlete's Ball*. Halifax: Novont Health Publishing, 2004.

McGill, Stuart. *Low Back Disorders: Evidence-Based Prevention and Rehabilitation*. Champaign, Ill.: Human Kinetics, 2002.

Nelson, Miriam and Sarah Wernick. *Strong Women, Strong Bones*. New York: Perigee, 2000.

Pilates, Joseph and William John Miller. *Return to Life through Contrology*. Incline Village, Nev.: Presentation Dynamics Inc., 1998.

Pilates, Joseph *Your Health*. Incline Village, Nev.: Presentation Dynamics Inc., 1998.

Posner-Mayer, Joanne. *Swiss Ball Applications for Orthopedic and Sports Medicine*. Longmont, Colo.: Ball Dynamics International, 1995.

Richardson, Carolyn, Gwendolen Jull, Julie Hides, and Paul Hodges. *Therapeutic Exercise for Spinal Segmental Stabilization in Low Back Pain*. London: Churchill Livingstone, 1999.

Robinson, Lynne and Gordon Thomson, *Body Control the Pilates Way*. London: Boxtree, 1997.

Rolf, Ida. *Rolfing*. Rochester, Vt.: Healing Arts Press, 1989.

Searle, Sally, and Cathy Meeus. *Secrets of Pilates*. New York: DK Publishing, 2001.

Siler, Brooke. *The Pilates Body*. New York: Broadway Books, 2000.

Spalding, Anne, Linda Kelly, Janet Santopietro, and Joanne Posner-Mayer. *Kids on the Ball*. Champaign, Ill.: Human Kinetics, 1999.

Stott-Merrithew, Moira and Beth Evans. *Comprehensive Matwork Manual*. Toronto: Merrithew Corporation, 2001.

Ungaro, Alycea. *Pilates Body in Motion*. New York: DK Publishing, 2002.

Winsor, Mari. *The Pilates Powerhouse*. Cambridge, Mass.: Perseus Books, 1999.

Videotapes/ DVDs

Colleen Craig's Pilates on the Ball. DVD/VHS/Color/45 mins. www.pilatesontheball.com

Exercises for the Pelvic Floor by Beate Carrière, VHS/Color/25 mins.

Fitball—Back to Functional Movement by Trish Scott, VHS/Color/30 mins.

Fitball—Upper Body Challenge; *Fitball—Lower Body Challenge* by Cheryl Soleway, VHS/Color/ 45mins each.

Pilates Mini-Ball Workout with Leslee Bender, VHS/Color.

Swiss Ball Applications for Orthopedic and Sports Medicine by Joanne Posner-Mayer, VHS/Color/90 mins.

Somarhythms by Ninoska Gómez, VHS/Color/12mins. Distributed by www.caboblancopark.com

The above videotapes and DVDs can be ordered through Ball Dynamics International; see the following page for contact information. *Colleen Craig's Pilates on the Ball* DVD and VHS can be ordered through Know Your Body Best in Canada and Ball Dynamics International in the United States.

Ball and Video Ordering Information

Ball Dynamics International, Inc.

Makers of Fitball®. Catalog of exercise balls, videotapes, and accessories. 800-752-2255. www.fitball.com

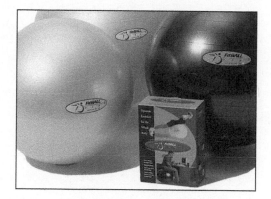

Know Your Body Best

Canadian distributor of exercise balls, *Colleen Craig's On the Ball* videotape and DVD, and, therapeutic massage equipment and supplies. 800-881-1681 (in Canada). www.knowyourbodybest.com

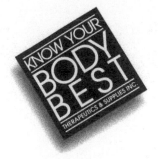

lululemon athletica

The mission of lululemon athletica is to increase health and personal success in our communities and in the world. lululemon.com—providing components for people to live longer, healthier, and more fun lives.

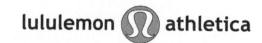

Acknowledgments

Two key pieces of luck have blessed my career. In 1997 I was introduced to Stott Pilates by Moira Stott-Merrithew, an outstanding Pilates teacher and director of what has now become one of the most important Pilates certification centers in the world. When I wasn't training with Moira, I worked with other talented teachers and colleagues: Beth Evans, Mariane Braaf, Syl Klotz, Elaine Biagi-Turner, Connie Di Salvo, Laura Helsel, and Danielle Belec. My luck in intercepting with all these outstanding teachers and colleagues at a time in my life when I was searching for a new direction astonishes me. The second piece of luck has to do with the intersection of my life with the ball. I am most grateful to Dayna Gutru, Gloria Miller, and their associates at Ball Dynamics International for supporting my work. I also want to thank Donna Micallef, Contance Rennett, the staff at Know Your Body Best in Toronto, and Dr. Nevio Cosani and the Cosani family in Italy.

I have had the good fortune of seeing the ball worked to tremendous advantage in many different places. Either in person, or through their books or tapes, the following exercise ball teachers and movement professionals have been instrumental in my understanding of the ball: Joanne Posner-Mayer, Ninoska Gómez, Rick Jemmett, Mari Naumovski, Cheryl Soleway, Trish Scott, Beate Carrière, and Paul Chek. Many people worked tirelessly to make sure my workshops abroad took off without a hitch and I would like to take this opportunity to thank them. In Italy: Paola del Fabbro and Enrico Ceron; in Zagreb: Asja Petersen, Rozi Dragicevic, and Sandra Ukalovic; in Hungary, Lajos Rozsavolgyi and his colleagues Mikail, Evette, Bea, and Eva; and in South Africa: Daniella Smoller of Thera Med and Christell Botes. Lately, I was reminded of an image I had of Poland before I made that trip: a dated vision of a rosy-cheeked woman with a kerchief tied at her chin. That in no way fitted with the participants in their designer sweats and sports bras, packing their oversized gym bags. Many thanks to Anita and Kamilla of Meden-Inmed for hosting the Warsaw and Krakow workshops and making sure ninety balls were blown up in the shortest time possible. Finally a warm thanks to my South American collegues: Maria Del Huerto Segura in Argentina and Renato Daher and Maira Antas in Brazil. Please invite me back soon.

I had never in my wildest dreams planned to make a career out of balls. My dreams for myself were about living in the world of books, not balls. Yet somehow my dreams have been realized, though not in the way I might have predicted. *Pilates on the Ball* is not only selling well but being translated into different languages! My second book, *Abs on the Ball*, is also being translated. I have no one to thank for these miracles but the tireless efforts of staff members at Healing Arts Press for successfully launching these books into the world. There would be no final product without Susan Davidson, my outstanding editor. Susan made the editing process on all three books painless—even enjoyable. Thanks to Peri Champine for creating the sensational covers, Jon Graham for believing (with Susan) in my work from the beginning, Jeanie Levitan for handling the endless details, and Rob Meadows and the rest of the design, production, and marketing teams at Healing Arts Press. I would also like to extend my thanks to Tara Persaud and Alan Zweig at Ten Speed Press and my agent, David Johnston.

Others have contributed to the completion of this book. Mari Naumovski of BodySpheres read the manuscript and gave much feedback; Claire Letemendia's expert editorial assistance greatly helped shape the manuscript; and physical therapist Dr. Miroslaw Kokosz supplied expertise and comment on this book. I am very grateful to Kevin Stoski, my nieces Lyndsey and Lauren Welch, and to my mother, Lorraine Craig, for agreeing to appear in the photos in this book. Thanks to Jody Stoski of Cinnamon Girl for the great makeup. Many thanks to David Scollard for his wonderful photography, Laraine Arsenault for the illustrations and preparing the artwork, and Robert Barnett for providing great additional images. Thanks to Russ Parker and Insiya Rasiwala of Lululemon Athletica for donating the beautiful clothing and yoga mats that appear in this book.

E-mails pour in weekly from teachers and students from around the world: unsolicited testimonials about what the ball means to them, how it has changed how they exercised, and how they taught others to exercise—thank you for your responses to this work. I am blessed with very loyal Toronto students and send them many, many thanks. Finally, I am most grateful for the steady, loving support of my friends and family, Laurie Colbert and Dominque Cardona for filming my video, and especially Lynne Viola (and Monty) for love and support over the years.

BOOKS OF RELATED INTEREST

Pilates on the Ball
The World's Most Popular Workout Using the Exercise Ball
by Colleen Craig

Abs on the Ball
A Pilates Approach to Building Superb Abdominals
by Colleen Craig

Trigger Point Therapy for Myofascial Pain
The Practice of Informed Touch
by Donna Finando, L.Ac., L.M.T., and Steven Finando, Ph.D., L.Ac.

Applied Kinesiology
Muscle Response in Diagnosis, Therapy, and Preventive Medicine
by Tom and Carole Valentine

The Five Tibetans
Five Dynamic Exercises for Health, Energy, and Personal Power
by Christopher S. Kilham

Thai Yoga Massage
A Dynamic Therapy for Physical Well-Being and Spiritual Energy
by Kam Thye Chow

Self-Awakening Yoga
The Expansion of Consciousness through the Body's Own Wisdom
by Don Stapleton, Ph.D.

Yoga on the Ball
Enhance Your Yoga Practice Using the Exercise Ball
by Carol Mitchell

Inner Traditions • Bear & Company
P.O. Box 388 • Rochester, VT 05767 • 1-800-246-8648
www.InnerTraditions.com

Or contact your local bookseller